PATIENT EDUCATION

Tools for Practice

Patient-Teaching Committee

Susan Baron, RN, BSN
Deborah Canty-Goodie, RN, BSN
Judith Clevesy Carleo, RN, BSN
Linda Donovan, RN, BSN
Ann Downey, RN, BSN, cochairman
Bonnie Marshall Edmonds, RN
Karen Esckilsen, RN, BSN
Melissa Flon, RN, BS
Jackie Gannon-Somerville, RN, BSN
Linda Goodman, RN, BSN, MSN

Georgette Hurrell, RN, BSN
Nora Koller, RN, BSN
Joan Krauss, RN, BSN
Nancy Leach, RN
Michelle McIntosh, RN, BSN, MSN
Carol Reilly, RN, BSN
Denise Richards, RN, BSN
Ginny Ryan-Morrell, RN
Karyl Woldum, RN, BSN, MSN, chairman

PATIENT EDUCATION

Tools for Practice

**Karyl M. Woldum
Kathleen A. Bower
Virginia Ryan-Morrell
Marilynn C. Towson
Karen S. Zander**

New England Medical
Center Hospitals
Boston

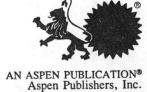
AN ASPEN PUBLICATION®
Aspen Publishers, Inc.
Rockville, Maryland
Royal Tunbridge Wells

Library of Congress Cataloging in Publication Data
Main entry under title:

Patient education.

"An Aspen publication."
Includes bibliographies.
1. Patient education—Handbooks, manuals, etc. 2. Nurse and patient—Handbooks, manuals, etc. 3. Health education—Handbooks, manuals, etc. 4. Lesson planning—Handbooks, manuals, etc. I. Woldum, Karyl M. [DNLM: 1. Patient Education—nurses' instruction. 2. Teaching—methods—nurscs' instruction. W 85 P2984]
RT90.P373   1985   610.73   84-20446
ISBN: 0-89443-563-9

Publisher: John R. Marozsan
Associate Publisher: Jack W. Knowles, Jr.
Editorial Director: N. Darlene Como
Executive Managing Editor: Margot G. Raphael
Managing Editor: M. Eileen Higgins
Editorial Services: Jane Coyle
Printing and Manufacturing: Debbie Collins

Library of Congress Catalog Card Number: 84-20446
ISBN: 0-89443-563-9

Printed in the United States of America

2 3 4 5

Table of Contents

Preface

One component of nursing that is universal to all areas of clinical practice is patient teaching. Nurses have accepted and enjoyed this role and have increased the professional literature with contributions on the rationale, content, and methodology for giving patients the information they need. However, with the growth of consumer pressure for informed consent and quality assurance, and with the JCAH requirements for providing proof that the "patient knowledge" outcome criteria are met, nurses are faced with the tasks of evaluating and documenting what is taught to patients. Because patient teaching involves a complex series of interactions between patient and nurse, documentation systems that reflect the teaching-learning process must be developed.

The Retrospective Audit Committee of the Department of Nursing, Tufts-New England Medical Center Hospital, began creating a system for documenting patient teaching more than eight years ago. We assessed our concurrent audits and found that the Problem-Oriented Medical Record (POMR) method of charting was too cumbersome for recording the detailed content of every teaching session. We sensed that patients were receiving unorganized facts from numerous well-meaning staff nurses or no information at all. Even with primary nursing it was unrealistic to expect one nurse in one session to teach patients everything they might need to know. We also realized that nurses would not use a system that was too elaborate, time consuming, or repetitious in addition to others already in use (Kardex, progress notes, flow sheets, to name a few). We could find no prototypes that would meet the needs of both pediatric and adult inpatient and ambulatory settings as well as fulfill all our requirements for comprehensive patient teaching.

Thus, through trial and error, we have developed a format and protocol for a system of documentation that encompasses (1) the patients' right to learn about their health care through individualized, organized communication with professional nurses, (2) nurses' need for knowledge in a handy reference that exceeds policies and procedures, (3) nurses' need for a useful documentation tool, and (4) the Retrospective Audit Committee's need for data confirming that specific outcome criteria have been met.

Because we were not experts in every field and because people tend to use what they make rather than what is handed them, we asked (with administrative backing) that personnel from each clinical area develop plans for the teaching they thought was most crucial. Each plan was edited for content and format and then added to the large collection of patient teaching plans then in use as part of patient medical records on a hospital-wide basis.

The teaching plans included in this book address many different kinds of learning needs. There are plans directed at the orientation of a patient to a unit, preparation for a diagnostic test, ability to perform self-care activities at home, and knowledge of diagnosis and treatment.

There are several general teaching plans whose use is directed to all patients or learning needs for which a specific plan is not available. They include the Primary Nursing, Medication, Preoperative, and Discharge teaching plans.

These patient teaching plans could never have been actualized without a supportive nursing administration. Administrative support enabled our group to put time and energy into the program and gave us the clout to make teaching part of a nurse's professional role.

We would like to recognize and thank Sandra Twyon, Chairman, Department of Nursing, for her assistance in establishing patient teaching as a priority. As you read the plans it will become clear why we want to express our special thanks to all the contributing registered nurses from every level of our organization. Finally, we must acknowledge the immeasurable contribution of Regina St. Cyr and Marie Gilarde, our secretaries, who prepared the manuscript.

Chapter 1

Teaching Plans

The teaching plans and guidelines included in this chapter are designed to be used by a registered nurse in any phase of a patient's education. They provide the nurse with a means to organize the presentation and to evaluate, by way of learner objectives, the patient's response. The teaching plans are designed to be used either in conjunction with problem-oriented charting or as an adjunct to other charting methods. A nurse, optimally the primary nurse, places a specific plan in the patient's progress notes as soon as the need for teaching is identified. Since plans are usually printed on colored paper, they can be easily located among the vast array of other data in the medical record. The checklist nature of the teaching plans facilitates rapid, accurate, and complete documentation. Content and objectives are signed off with the date and the registered nurse's initials, giving their completion the same legality as the patient's medication record. Besides fostering accountability, the checklist format also encourages follow-through when teaching has begun in one unit and the patient is either transferred to another unit or discharged to an ambulatory clinic or to the Visiting Nurse Association for follow-up care. There is also space for the nurses to write an overall evaluation of the patient's movement toward meeting the objectives.

Guidelines to enable the nurse to teach more effectively and evaluate the sessions are included with some of the plans in this book. They are organized to correlate with the learner objectives of the teaching plans to facilitate their use as a reference and have been a valuable asset for new or inexperienced nurses. In our setting we have found it useful to provide each nursing unit with a complete notebook of sample plans and guidelines. Each unit also has a stock of plans that are most frequently used, and a mechanism for ordering necessary plans is worked out through unit coordination.

In addition to the plans and guidelines, handouts have been developed for patients and their families' use on discharge or between clinic visits. Handouts can further enhance teaching that may already be completed. They ensure that regardless of how well patients and their significant other met the learner objectives, they have reliable information when they are away from the immediate hospital environment. Handouts are included in this book.

The existence of these teaching plans demonstrates that it is possible to formalize a system for documenting patient teaching and for standardizing the content. Teaching plans and guidelines must be consistent with standards of care but flexible enough to be used by any nurse in individualizing the content and methodology for a specific patient. These plans were designed to concur with the methods of care and types of patients in one institution. It is probably impossible to begin using them in other agencies without revision according to the level of acuteness of patients' conditions, the level of nursing knowledge, and each agency's policies and standards. This is by no means an all-inclusive collection—many subjects not included here may be vital to other institutions. The results from retrospective auditing were our stimulus for these plans—your motivation may be different. We offer these examples as encouragement to those considering the development of a practical, no-frills system of patient education.

UTILIZING THE TEACHING PLAN

To assist the nurse in documenting teaching and its results, the patient teaching form has three columns that must be signed with the date and the nurse's signature as content is delivered and reinforced and as the patient meets the behavioral objectives (Exhibit 1).

Column 1 includes content and reinforcement delivered, with the date and a registered nurse's signature. As the nurse presents and reinforces the content material to the patient, the date and nurse's signature are recorded opposite the specific content described.

Column 2 includes the learner objective met, the date, and a registered nurse's signature. When the patient satisfactorily meets each objective, the date and the nurse's signature are recorded opposite the specific objective.

Column 3, designated not applicable, is provided for recording those objectives and content that do not apply specifically to the teaching plan.

EVALUATION

At the conclusion of the teaching process or the patient's discharge from the health care setting, the nurse must summarize and evaluate the effectiveness of teaching. This evaluation should reflect the patient's ability to meet the objectives of the teaching plan and the quality of the learning: Was the patient able to learn only the basic components of the plan covered? The nurse's evaluation will aid other health providers if it also describes the pace of teaching most appropriate for this patient and the methods and approaches found most beneficial. Of equal importance is the identification of those objectives that the patient was unable to accomplish and the nurse's plan to correct these learning deficiencies. The plan for follow-up might include a referral to a visiting nurse association or contact with the nurse who will see the patient in an outpatient setting to continue teaching.

Exhibit 1 A Sample Teaching Plan

	Content/ Reinforcement Delivered Date & RN	Learner Objectives Met Date & RN	Not Applicable

SEIZURE
 	
Purpose
 	
To teach the patient with seizures and the family the characteristics of a seizure disorder and its management at home.
 	
Content
 	
    I. Definition of a seizure
   II. Description of characteristics of the patient's seizure
 III. Management of the patient during and after a seizure
 IV. Anticonvulsant medications
  V. Safety measures at home
 VI. Reasons to notify the physician
VII. Follow-up
	1/24/84 J.Smith RN
	1/24/84 J.Smith RN
	{ 1/25/84 S.CLARK RN
	{ 1/26/84 J.Smith RN
	1/26/84 J.Smith RN
	1/27/84 J.Smith RN
	1/27/84 J.Smith RN
	1/27/84 J.Smith RN		

Learner Objectives I. The patient and significant other describe a seizure in simple terms and identify the specific seizure disorder. _____ _____			

A. The patient and family state that a seizure is a symptom of a disturbance of nervous system function that may be caused by trauma, infection, fever, metabolic disorder, drug intoxication, or unknown cause.
   B. The patient and family state the seizure type:
     1. Grand mal
     2. Petit mal
     3. Febrile
     4. Abstinence
     5. Focal
     6. Other _____
		1/24/84
		J. Smith RN
		
		1/24/84
		J. Smith RN	

II. The patient and family describe the characteristics of the patient's type of seizure.
   A. Loss of consciousness
   B. Body twitching
   C. Aura
   D. Incontinence
   E. Eyes deviated to side
   F. Staring spells
		1/24/84
		J.Smith RN
		1/25/84
		S. CLARK RN	

Exhibit 1 continued

	Content/ Reinforcement Delivered Date & RN	Learner Objectives Met Date & RN	Not Applicable
G. Vomiting or foaming at mouth			
H. Incoherence			
I. Postictal stage			
J. Other _____			
III. The patient and family state management during seizure activity.		1/25/84 S. CLARK RN	
A. Remain with patient during seizure.		1/25/84 S.CLARK RN	
B. Observe duration and describe seizure.		1/25/84 S.CLARK RN	
C. Do not try to stop seizure by slapping face or giving medications.		1/25/84 S.CLARK RN	
D. Do not physically restrain patient.		1/25/84 S.CLARK RN	
E. Protect patient from self-injury by turning head and body to the side and place a soft object under the head.		1/25/84 S.CLARK RN	
F. Do not put hard objects into the mouth. The patient will not "swallow" the tongue when the head is turned to the side.			
G. If patient is turning blue, clear the airway and give mouth-to-mouth breathing.		1/26/84 J. Smith RN	
H. During postictal state, patient will be tired and may complain of headache, restlessness, or muscle weakness.			
I. Other _____			
IV. The patient and family describe anticonvulsant medication and meet objectives of medication teaching guide.		1/26/84 J. Smith RN (may need more reinforcement)	
V. The patient and family state safety measures.		1/27/84 J. Smith RN	
A. If child, do not leave unattended in high chair.			N/A
B. If child, keep bed and play area free of hard objects to protect from harm.			N/A
C. Activity is not restricted but caution should be taken in high areas, during gymnastics, in work area, and while swimming.		1/27/84 J. Smith RN	
D. Patient is to wear medic alert identification.		1/27/84 J.Smith RN	
E. Work and school nurse should know of patient's seizure disorder.		1/27/84 J.Smith RN	
F. If patient has aura, patient should seek privacy and safe place to lie down before seizure if possible.			
G. Automobile licensure is regulated by states. Inquire about rules for seizure patient through registry of motor vehicles.			
H. Work position should be evaluated for safety regulations, e.g., high construction area.			

Exhibit 1 continued

	Content/ Reinforcement Delivered Date & RN	Learner Objectives Met Date & RN	Not Applicable
VI. Patient and family state when to contact physician. A. Seizure activity persists or there is increased frequency. B. Patient is unable to take medication. C. Other *Out of medication* VII. The patient and family describe follow-up care. A. A record of seizures noting date, time, and description of seizures should be kept. B. Support system is available through epilepsy society. C. Follow-up appointment *2/10/84* D. Physician #: *488-2642* Emergency room #: *424-5000*		1/27/84 J. Smith RN 1/27/84 J. Smith RN 1/27/84 J. Smith RN 1/27/84 J. Smith RN	

Evaluation

If patient or significant others are unable to complete some or all of this teaching plan, document evaluation in progress notes.

Mr. Keep was very interested in learning about his newly diagnosed seizure disorder. His wife also participated in teaching sessions. This gentleman was able to comprehend the nature of his problem and move quickly to learning how to manage at home. Mr. Keep will need additional reinforcement about safety measures and medication. His wife needs more instruction about how to protect him during a seizure. I have contacted M. Sweat RN, neurology outpatient nurse to continue instruction.

Joan Smith RN

Part I

The Cardiovascular System

	Content/ Reinforcement Delivered	Learner Objectives Met	Not Applicable
	Date & RN	Date & RN	

ANGINA

Purpose

To give information to the patient and family about the causes of angina, recognition of the symptoms of angina, and steps to take to relieve symptoms.

Content

- I. Anatomy and physiology of the heart
  - A. Muscle
  - B. Blood vessels
- II. Pathophysiology of angina
  - A. Atherosclerosis
  - B. Spasm
  - C. Cause
- III. Symptoms of angina
- IV. Risk factors related to angina
- V. Situations that may precipitate anginal episodes
- VI. Home treatment of an angina episode
- VII. Care of nitroglycerin prescription
- VIII. Reasons to contact physician
- IX. Follow-up

Learner Objectives

- I. The patient describes in simple terms the anatomy and physiology of the heart muscle and blood vessels.
  - A. The heart muscle is a strong hollow organ that acts as a pump. It pumps blood throughout the body and lungs.
  - B. The coronary blood vessels surround the heart and feed the heart muscle with blood containing oxygen and nutrients.
- II. The patient states in simple terms the definition and causes of angina.
  - A. Angina is the discomfort caused by a decrease in the amount of blood feeding the heart muscle.
  - B. Angina is a signal that there is temporary poor circulation to the muscle.
  - C. The cause of angina may either be a buildup of fatty substances (cholesterol) on the lining of the blood vessels that feed the heart, or a sudden spasm of the blood vessels causing a slowing or stoppage of blood supply or both.
- III. The patient states the most common symptoms of angina:
  - A. Chest or arm discomfort (tightness, squeezing, aching)
  - B. Indigestion
  - C. Aching that is felt in the neck, jaw, throat, shoulder, or back
  - D. Breathlessness, weakness, sweating, dizziness
  - E. My own symptoms are _____

	Content/ Reinforcement Delivered Date & RN	Learner Objectives Met Date & RN	Not Applicable

IV. The patient defines risk factors and describes the controllable and uncontrollable risk factors.
   A. Risk factors are habits or characteristics that increase the probability of developing a narrowing of the blood vessels that feed the heart muscle.
   B. Controllable factors are
     1. Cigarette smoking
     2. High blood pressure
     3. Increased amount of fatty substance in blood
     4. Stress or tension
     5. Lack of exercise
     6. Obesity
   C. Uncontrollable factors are
     1. Diabetes
     2. Family history
     3. Males and persons over the age of 50
   D. Patient's risk factors
     Controllable
 	
     _____
     _____
     _____
 	
     Uncontrollable
 	
     _____
     _____
     _____
 	
V. The patient states the situations that may precipitate an anginal episode:
   A. Sudden outbursts of activity or emotion, since they place unusual demands on the heart and increase its consumption of oxygen
   B. Heavy lifting such as picking up children, grocery bags, suitcases
   C. Activities such as stair climbing, prolonged walking, and sexual activity, which may overexert the heart
   D. Extreme temperature changes such as being out in cold or hot weather or showering in extreme hot or cold water
   E. Constipation with accompanied straining, which can cause an increased workload on the heart
   F. The patient's anginal attacks precipitated by the following:
 	
     _____
     _____
     _____
 	
VI. The patient states the home treatment of anginal episodes.
   A. When the anginal episode begins, stop what I am doing.			

	Content/ Reinforcement Delivered	Learner Objectives Met	Not Applicable
	Date & RN	Date & RN	

B. Place nitroglycerin tablet under the tongue. Note the time.

C. If discomfort is not relieved, take another tablet under the tongue 5 minutes after the first.

D. Up to three tablets may be used, each 5 minutes apart, for each anginal episode.

E. If discomfort is unrelieved, go to the nearest emergency room.

F. After the discomfort is relieved, resume usual activity.

VII. The patient states the care of nitroglycerin prescription.

  A. Nitroglycerin must be refilled every 4 to 6 months once the presciption has been opened.

  B. If nitroglycerin is fresh, it will burn or tingle under the tongue.

  C. It must be kept cool and in a dark container.

  D. A supply of tablets must be kept with the patient at all times.

VIII. The patient states reasons to contact the physician or go to the emergency room:

  A. An angina episode not relieved after taking nitroglycerin

  B. Angina episodes occurring at rest

  C. Increasing severity of angina episode

  D. Increasing frequency of angina episodes

IX. The patient describes follow-up:

Clinic physician #: _____

Local physician #: _____

Emergency room #: _____

Evaluation

If patient or significant others are unable to complete some or all of this teaching plan, document evaluation in progress notes.

	Content/ Reinforcement Delivered Date & RN	Learner Objectives Met Date & RN	Not Applicable

HOME CARE FOR THE ADULT HEMATOLOGY AND ONCOLOGY PATIENT
 	
Purpose
 	
To maintain the patient in the highest level of wellness and assist the patient in assuming responsibilities for self-care.
 	
Content
 	
    I. Description of condition in simple terms
   II. Description of the signs and symptoms of a bleed and the means of prevention
 III. Description of signs and symptoms of infection and means of prevention
 IV. Description of the signs and symptoms of anemia and means of prevention
   V. Activities of daily living
 VI. Description of the signs and symptoms of inappropriate psychological coping and means of prevention
VII. Description of signs and symptoms of central nervous system involvement
VIII. Content of medication teaching plan on following medications: _____
 IX. Description of how to contact primary care team 24 hours a day
  X. Description of prescribed diet and normal weight
 XI. Health maintenance
XII. Follow-up			

Learner Objectives
 	
   I. The patient describes the problem in simple terms.
 	
_____
 	
_____
 	
  II. The patient reports signs and symptoms of bleeding and means of prevention.
    A. The patient states the signs and symptoms of a major bleed are black or bloody stools, bleeding from cut or nose lasting more than 30 minutes, dizziness, headache, shortness of breath, paroxysmal nocturnal dyspnea, orthopnea, blackouts, irritability, listlessness, pulse above normal, red urine, or bruising.
    B. The patient states that a major bleed is prevented when platelets are less than 20,000 by avoiding rectal inserts, invasive procedures, ASA-containing products, and contact sports. Patient will report all trauma, especially			

	Content/ Reinforcement Delivered Date & RN	Learner Objectives Met Date & RN	Not Applicable

head trauma. Lubricate mucous membranes, especially during intercourse. Use a soft toothbrush.

III. The patient reports signs and symptoms of infections and means of prevention.

  A. Upper respiratory infection
    1. The patient states that the signs and symptoms of an upper respiratory infection (URI) are fever, cough, shaking chills, green or yellow sputum, chest pain, sore throat, earache, and sinus pain.
    2. The patient states that complications of URI are prevented when white blood cells are low by taking a temperature every 4 hours and avoiding persons with URI or infectious diseases such as chicken pox, measles, and mumps.

  B. Monilia
    1. The patient states that the signs and symptoms of monilia are white patches, ulcers in the mouth, and vaginal discharge.
    2. The patient states that monilia can be prevented or detected early by inspecting for monilia every day and frequently rinsing with equal parts of water and peroxide.

  C. Urinary tract infection
    1. The patient states that the signs and symptoms of a urinary tract infection are pain on urination, belly or back pain, hesitancy, frequency, retention, bloody urine, and fever.
    2. The patient states that urinary tract infections can be prevented by females washing the perineum from front to back, maintaining fluids at 2 quarts a day, and emptying the bladder before and after intercourse.

  D. Rectal abscess
    1. The patient states the signs and symptoms of a rectal abscess are rectal discharge, bleeding, or pain.
    2. The patient states that a rectal abscess is prevented by avoiding rectal inserts during periods of low white blood cell counts.

  E. Infected wounds
    1. The patient states that the signs and symptoms of an infected cut are swelling, discharge, pain, redness, or warmth.
    2. The patient states that the skin should be inspected daily and invasive procedures avoided during periods of low white blood cell counts.

	Content/ Reinforcement Delivered Date & RN	Learner Objectives Met Date & RN	Not Applicable
F. The patient states that the signs and symptoms of a bowel complication are changes in bowel habits lasting more than 2 days.			
IV. The patient reports the signs and symptoms of anemia and means of prevention.			
A. The patient states that the signs and symptoms of anemia are fatigue, pallor, shortness of breath, paroxysmal nocturnal dyspnea, orthopnea, dizziness, palpitations, and pedal enema.			
B. The patient states that during periods of anemia, rest periods are planned between activities, rising from lying is done gradually, and activity is stopped when symptoms increase.			
V. The patient discusses activities of daily living.			
A. The patient lists activities of daily living (ADL) that can be performed.			
B. The patient states that it is necessary to report any changes in the ability to perform ADL.			
C. The patient lists interventions to be taken when ADL cannot be performed.			
VI. The patient reports signs and symptoms of inappropriate psychological coping and means of prevention.			
A. The patient states that the signs and symptoms of inappropriate psychological coping are functioning poorly at school or work, change in personality (withdrawal) or irritability, insomnia or nightmares.			
B. The patient states that coping is better achieved by verbalizing openly to the medical team and among family members, talking together with medical staff and family, dealing directly and honestly with questions about death, family counseling, maintaining normal life patterns, and setting normal limits and discipline with both parents and children.			
VII. The patient states that the signs and symptoms of central nervous symptom involvement are headache, dizziness, projectile vomiting, ataxia, and blurred vision.			
VIII. The patient completes the teaching plan on the following medications: _____.			
IX. The patient states how to contact the primary care team 24 hours a day.			
X. The patient describes a balanced or prescribed diet, weighs self every day, and calls in a weight gain or loss.			
XI. The patient lists health maintenance needs. It is safest to have procedures done during remission (ophthalmology, dental, self-breast exam, gynecology, immunization, minor surgery). Otherwise the patient should check with the physician.			

	Content/ Reinforcement Delivered	Learner Objectives Met	Not Applicable
	Date & RN	Date & RN	
XII. The patient states how to make and check for a follow-up appointment before leaving from hospitalization or ambulatory visit.			
Evaluation			
If patient or significant others are unable to complete some or all of this teaching plan, document evaluation in progress notes.			

GUIDELINES: HOME CARE FOR THE ADULT HEMATOLOGY AND ONCOLOGY PATIENT

Aim of Nursing

To maintain the highest level of wellness and assist the patient in assuming responsibility for self-care.

Specifically the content addresses patients receiving chemotherapy for solid and liquid tumors.

I. Patient describes the condition in simple terms, for example:

    A. Patients with leukemia usually describe their disease as the body producing a large amount of abnormal white cells that do not work well (to fight infection) and can interfere by crowding the bone marrow, spleen, and lymph nodes.

    B. Patient with solid tumors can state the name of the tumor and where the tumor is located. Relate why the patient is experiencing symptoms; i.e., increased lymph nodes in the axilla will cause the arm to swell; increased spleen can press on stomach and produce anorexia; lung cancer will cause coughing.

    C. Due to the fact that the medical staff often discusses blood count values, it is helpful that the patients know that the blood is composed of three elements:

        Red blood cells (hematocrit and hemoglobin) that carry oxygen. When these are low, the condition is called *anemia.*

        White blood cells (white count and differential) that fight infection. Specifically, polycytes (polys) fight bacteria, and lymphocytes fight virus.

        Platelets prevent bleeding by clotting at the sight of a bleed.

    D. The patient should know the terms *relapse* and *remission*:

        1. *Remission.* Blast cells (the primitive abnormal white cells) or tumor cells are destroyed by chemotherapy. A patient in remission can enjoy unlimited activity, can attend school or work, and should be treated as a healthy person and be allowed to follow a normal life routine.

        2. *Relapse.* The reappearance of abnormal cell or tumor in bone marrow, peripheral blood, or x-ray. Precautions for activity are outlined under complications.

	Content/ Reinforcement Delivered Date & RN	Learner Objectives Met Date & RN	Not Applicable

PATIENTS RECEIVING RADIATION TO THE HEAD AND NECK

Purpose

To determine the patient's concept of the illness and understanding of radiation therapy.

To assess the patient's knowledge of the total therapy plan.

To give specific information regarding radiation therapy to the head and neck as it applies to the patient's condition.

To inform the patient about side effects specific to the individual therapy and how they can be minimized as well as the importance of oral and dental care and good nutrition.

To make the patient aware of the consequences of noncompliance with treatment as it applies to comfort and health.

Content

  I. Review of general radiotherapy teaching plan and description of the treatment
 II. Description of treatment area
III. Side effects specific to head and neck radiation therapy
 IV. Skin care
  V. Care of mucous membrane
 VI. Dietary adjustments
VII. Restrictions in activities of daily living

Learner Objectives

  I. The patient describes general radiotherapy points and personal treatment plan.
 II. The patient describes the area of the tumor, the location of any enlarged nodes, the treatment area, and the sequence and timing of therapy.
III. The patient describes the expected side effects.
 IV. The patient describes the care of the skin during and after radiation therapy.
  V. The patient describes methods used to relieve the side effects of radiation on the mucous membrane.
 VI. The patient describes dietary adjustments and methods that can be used to make eating more comfortable.
VII. The patient states the restrictions in activities of daily living, as well as the consequences of noncompliance with the treatment regimen.

Evaluation

If patient or significant others are unable to complete some or all of this teaching plan, document evaluation in progress notes.

GUIDELINES: PATIENTS RECEIVING RADIATION TO THE HEAD AND NECK

Background information for the nurse: This plan deals only with problems related to radiation of tumors within the oral cavity, pharynx, larynx, nose, and paranasal sinuses. In general, tumors of the head and neck constitute a regional problem; that is, they remain confined to this area and metastasize to distant sites only very late in their evolution. Tumors in certain areas may be highly curable, yet the same cancer metastasized to the neck nodes may not be controlled by radiation.

The following types of persons are more prone to problems in these areas:

1. Alcoholics and heavy drinkers
2. Smokers and users of tobacco products
3. Those who have poor oral hygiene and insufficient dental care
4. Workers whose occupation involves the use of an irritating or toxic substance

The treatment of cancers of the head and neck often combines two types of therapy, i.e., surgery and radiotherapy. The radiation may be preoperative or postoperative, depending on the tumor, location, and extent of surgery required. Chemotherapy is not usually effective in treatment of these lesions, but it may be used as adjunctive therapy for metastasis.

I. Patient completes objective I of the general radiotherapy teaching plan.
II. The patient describes the area of the tumor, the location of any enlarged nodes, the treatment area, and the sequence and timing of therapy. When describing the treatment area to the patient, the nurse needs to be aware of the structures involved by the disease and the location of the enlarged neck or supraclavicular nodes. The involved areas and treatment plan may be obtained from the patient's physician. Figure 1 indicates the general treatment areas.
III. The patient describes the side effects that can be expected from treatment. All patients receiving radi-

Figure 1 Treatment Areas of the Head and Neck

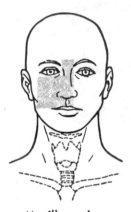

Maxillary sinus

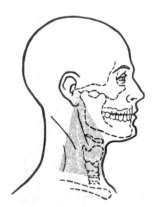

Lateral neck node

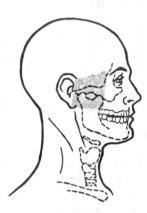

Nasopharynx

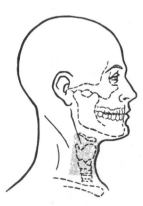

Larynx

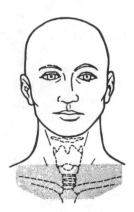

Supraclavicular nodes

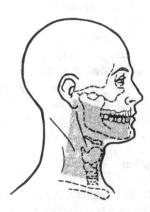

Base of tongue

ation to the head and neck do not have the same side effects. The severity of the reaction differs, depending on the dosage and placement of treatment portals.

A. Mucous membrane reactions
1. Mucositis or radioepithelitis. These describe inflammation of the mucosa. The epithelium of the mucosa begins to react in about 1½ to 2 weeks. It can react sooner as a result of irritation such as smoking or a large amount of hard liquor. Desquamation, a sloughing of the mucosa, occurs in about 2 to 3 weeks. The tissue never completely recovers, yet the reaction is termed reversible. When the dosage reaches 3,000 to 4,000 rads in 3 to 4 weeks, the reaction is acute. Capillary congestion causes the deep red coloring of the mucosa, and it persists even after desquamation.

   The classic characteristics of inflammation apply to mucositis. The patient complains of redness, swelling, heat, and tenderness of the mucosal tissue. When mucositis occurs in the oral cavity, soreness is the primary complaint; in the pharynx, dysphagia; and in the larynx, hoarseness.
2. Dryness of the mouth. In the process of radiating the oral cavity, major salivary glands and small mucous glands sustain damage. This usually begins in the first few weeks of treatment, and the severity is determined by time and dosage. The quality and quantity of saliva are altered. The serous portion of the saliva is diminished considerably, and the mucous portion is lessened and thickened. The actual dryness does not begin until later in the treatment. This creates a bothersome situation for the patient and is a prime complaint during and after treatment. If the treatment has been radical and has included the major glands, the problem will last for many months, and the quantity of saliva will not usually return to a normal level. The patient may need to drink with all meals to assist in swallowing and may want to carry a container of liquid at all times to relieve unusual dryness.
3. Dental changes. The changes in the mucosa have greater implications for patients who have their natural teeth. Normal saliva assists in preventing caries, but the thick, sticky saliva that results from radiation is no longer effective. Therefore caries can occur during radiation and often shortly after treatment has finished. This problem is serious because

tooth extractions from an irradiated jaw may induce osteonecrosis. To prevent this, all patients are given a dental checkup before irradiation. All teeth that might require extraction within 2 years are removed and the remainder repaired. The patient then must have instruction and supervision in oral care. Good oral care habits and constant dental attention must be maintained throughout the patient's lifetime.
4. Taste changes. Patients may complain of a "terrible" or "tinny" taste in the mouth. Acid foods seem to cause a disagreeable metallic sensation. Patients also complain that their favorite foods, even water, do not taste good and that efforts by their families to provide a tasty dish are wasted. This is generally a temporary problem, but it can last several months. This taste may be due partially to changes in pH of saliva.
5. Dysphagia. When the pharynx is in the field of radiation, the mucositis and desquamation cause dysphagia. It may fluctuate as the tumor decreases in size but worsen as the dosage of radiation accumulates. The degree of severity indicates what must be done to alleviate it or to prevent other problems. When dysphagia occurs, patients are instructed to continue an adequate nutritional intake by including more soft foods or increasing liquid foods, even using a dietary supplement if necessary.
6. Hoarseness. Tumors on or between the vocal cords may interfere with their vibrations and cause hoarseness. It is an early symptom and may be present at the patient's initial visit. During treatment the degree of hoarseness may vary. If the tumor decreases in size, the voice may improve. When the epithelial reaction peaks, the hoarseness may worsen. In most cases this situation improves when treatment terminates or shortly thereafter, but it may last many months.
7. Dryness of nasopharynx. When the nasal passages or the frontal sinuses are radiated, the reaction is the same as that for the oral mucosa. The patient will have dryness and a "stuffed nose" or a feeling of getting a head cold.

B. Complications of radiotherapy. Fungal infections may resemble certain aspects of a radiation reaction but should not be confused with it. Why fungal infections occur is not known definitely, but in some instances they may be influenced by the following:

1. Altered pH of the saliva
2. Poor physical health
3. Insufficient nutritional intake

IV. The patient describes the care of the skin during and after radiation therapy.
   A. In shaving, the patient must use an electric razor and shave dry. For the following reasons conventional shaving must be avoided:
      1. Lather is a soap; it is an irritant and would increase the reaction.
      2. The patient increases the chance of cutting and nicking the skin, which could become infected and necessitate a break in treatment.
      3. Lotions used before and after shaving are to be avoided, since they also act as irritants.
   B. Women should not use depilatories, bleaching agents, dyes, or makeup within the treated area.
   C. The patient should avoid rough clothing against the treatment area to prevent abrasion.
   D. Prolonged exposure of the treatment area to sunlight is to be avoided lifelong. A hat with a brim or a scarf may be sufficient protection, depending on the treated area.

V. Patient describes the methods used to relieve the side effects of radiation to the mucous membranes:
   A. Mucositis or radioepithelitis. The mucosa must be observed at least weekly; if the patient complains of oral discomfort, the complaint should be investigated. Mucositis can occur without comparable reddening of the outer skin, causing the patient great discomfort and possible bleeding of oral tissues. When acute mucositis occurs, the treatment may be as follows:
      1. Possible rest from radiotherapy for a few days
      2. Xylocaine viscous gargle for comfort
      3. Anesthetic lozenges for comfort
      4. Lavage, with at least 1 quart of saline and soda bicarbonate solution three times a day and preferably more often for cleaning and comfort
      5. Analgesics if necessary
   B. Dryness of the mouth. To alleviate this problem, patients are encouraged to use lavage three or more times a day. For edentulous patients, candy or gum may be helpful; for persons with natural teeth, sugar-free products should be used. If the dryness interferes with their ability to chew and swallow, the food should be moistened with gravies or natural juices. Patients are also encouraged to take a sip of liquid to help them swallow. Lemon-glycerine swabs or a homemade solution may be used to give gentle oral care. Patients sometimes find one particular liquid that helps them more than others. Some patients carry a container of water with them constantly. Increasing the humidity of the home by using a room humidifier or putting containers of water on radiators is also helpful. Saliva substitutes are now available, and some of these are more effective than others (personal preference may play a part in this).

To prevent dental caries, patients are to brush the teeth gently after each meal and at bedtime, avoiding irritation to the gums. Lavage should be done after brushing. Toothpaste is not recommended during treatment because it can be very irritating to oral tissues.

Fluoride "trays" are plastic molds that are made to fit over a patient's teeth. They become a lifetime, integral part of daily oral care. The trays are filled with fluoride gel and snapped on over the teeth. They are to be used 10 minutes daily. It is believed that the use of this method will decrease dental caries. When the fluoride trays are made for the patient, it is important to remind the patient to check on where and how to replenish the supply of fluoride. It can be expensive; therefore the patient should investigate the sources available before fluoride is used up.
   C. Hoarseness. For relief of hoarseness, the patient must use the voice as little as possible. This also helps prevent long-range problems from straining the voice. Symptomatic relief may be obtained from the following:
      1. Lavage
      2. Oral anesthetic agents
      3. Lozenges
   D. Dryness of nasopharynx. Symptomatic relief of dryness may be obtained by:
      1. Lavage of nasopharynx with a nasal douche or by nasal spray with a saline solution (the spray must be used often or for a few minutes at each treatment to wash tissue with sufficient solution to give relief)
      2. Increased humidity of home or immediate living area

VI. Patient states dietary adjustments and methods used to make eating more comfortable:
   A. Taste changes. There is not much help for taste changes except time, but patients are encouraged to do the following:
      1. Lavage.
      2. Avoid acidic foods or foods that they find to be unpleasant until the symptoms disappear.
      3. Avoid highly seasoned foods.
   B. Dysphagia. To alleviate this problem and the additional difficulties that it can cause, some of the following methods might be used, depending

on the length of time the difficulty exists, its severity, and the physician's preference.

1. Lavage to help alleviate other side effects (dryness of mucous membrane) that can contribute to dysphagia.

2. Gargle with an anesthetic that may also be swallowed, i.e., Dyclone or viscous xylocaine.

   Caution: Patients may lose their gag reflex after ingestion. Care should be taken when the patient eats or drinks within 60 minutes after its use.

For the nurse: It is important that the patient maintain adequate fluid intake. If this is not possible, other forms of intervention must be considered by the physician, i.e., intravenous therapy and nasogastric tube feeding.

VII. Patient states the restrictions in activities of daily living, as well as the consequences of noncompliance with the treatment regimen:

A. Restrictions
   1. No smoking
   2. No alcoholic beverages or commercial mouthwashes
   3. No prosthetics in treatment area, i.e., dentures
   4. No rough clothing against the skin
   5. Avoidance of prolonged direct sunlight
   6. Daily treatment attendance except for illness or bad weather
   7. Frequent mouth care
   8. Healthful diet

B. Consequences of noncompliance
   1. Increased erythema and discomfort
   2. Formation of ulcerations
   3. Prolonged healing

4. Increased length of time for treatments
5. Weakness and ill health

For the nurse: Often patients who come for radiation of the head and neck have other special needs. These patients need adjustments in the usual teaching methods to assist them in obtaining maximum benefits from the treatment. The nurse must observe the patient physically, mentally, and emotionally to assess what the person is capable of doing for oneself, to evaluate what help is available, and to do the necessary teaching with the helper. For instance, the patient can be instructed to gargle and swish the oral lavage solution from a glass if unable to manipulate the lavage bag. At least 3 quarts of solution should be used each day.

When teaching nasal care to a patient who is not mentally aware or in good muscular control, avoid nasal lavage, because breathing must be coordinated with the lavage to prevent aspiration. Rather than risk aspiration, nasal spray atomizers or nasal spray–type bottles that have been filled with normal saline and soda bicarbonate solution should be used and the patient instructed to use this as often as desired. Humidification of the immediate environment helps as well, especially at night.

Some patients have tracheotomies or laryngectomies for varying lengths of time. The patient's ability to care for these areas must be reviewed, and in some cases a total teaching plan might even be prepared. Additional teaching time and supervision at home could be provided by a visiting nurse association referral. The nurse must assess any changes in the patient's condition and make the patient aware of available services, i.e., speech clinics or speaking devices, alcohol treatment services, and rental equipment for special problems.

	Content/ Reinforcement Delivered Date & RN	Learner Objectives Met Date & RN	Not Applicable

HYPERTENSION
 	
Purpose
 	
To increase patient and family knowledge of hypertension through discussion of causative factors, symptoms, and complication of untreated hypertension.
To increase adherence to health regimen.
To support patient and family role in blood pressure treatment through discussion of life style modification, individual cardiovascular risk profile, and specific pharmacologic treatment.
 	
Content
 	
   I. Brief discussion of physiology of normal blood pressure versus hypertension
  II. Definition of hypertension as an asymptomatic disease and, in most patients, a disease of unknown etiology
 III. Discussion of the relationship of untreated hypertension to organ disease
 IV. Discussion of signs and symptoms of complications of high blood pressure
  V. Description of diet and life style modifications in the context of individual cardiovascular risk profile
 VI. Discussion of specific antihypertensive medication
    A. Uses
    B. Action
    C. Side effects
 VII. Demonstration of home equipment, when applicable
VIII. Follow-up			

Learner Objectives
 	
  I. The patient describes the normal physiology of blood pressure.
    A. Blood pressure is defined as the force required to circulate the blood throughout the body. The heart is the pump that creates this force.
    B. The two numbers in the blood pressure represent the pressure exerted against the blood vessel walls while the heart is contracting (systole) and the pressure while the heart is at rest (diastole).
    C. Although there is no absolute dividing line between normal and high blood pressure, blood pressures below 140/90 are usually considered to be in the normal range.
 II. The patient defines hypertension.			

	Content/ Reinforcement Delivered Date & RN	Learner Objectives Met Date & RN	Not Applicable
III. The patient describes the risks of untreated hypertension. High blood pressure imposes an extra burden on the heart and blood vessels. When the heart pumps against an abnormally high pressure for a long period of time, the walls of the heart thicken and the heart itself enlarges. High blood pressure can eventually damage the blood vessels in the kidneys and in the brain, leading to kidney failure and stroke.			
IV. The patient states signs and symptoms of complications of uncontrollable high blood pressure and states that if they occur, the patient will notify the physician: A. Severe headache B. Dizziness C. Weakness in an arm or leg D. Sudden visual change E. Chest pain F. Shortness of breath			

V. The patient describes the specific antihypertensive treatment including diet, life-style changes, and medication.
A. Treatment for hypertension depends on the level of blood pressure as well as many other factors such as
  1. Age
  2. Race
  3. Sex
  4. Family history
  5. Cholesterol level
  6. Diabetes
  7. Cigarette smoking
  8. Alcohol intake
  9. Birth control pills
B. In 90% of cases, hypertension is a disease that can be treated and not cured.
C. Recommended changes in life style include the following:
  1. Cutting down on the amount of salt in the diet. Salt intake increases the total amount of fluid in the vessels, thus contributing to elevated blood pressure.
  2. Losing weight if overweight because studies show that significant weight loss can help to control blood pressure.
  3. Stopping smoking.
  4. Drinking alcohol only in moderate amounts (less than 2 ounces daily).
  5. Exercise, with approval from the doctor.			

	Content/ Reinforcement Delivered Date & RN	Learner Objectives Met Date & RN	Not Applicable
VI. The patient meets the objectives of the medication teaching plan for each medication presented, discusses, and emphasizes that it is important to 　A. Take the medication regularly as directed 　B. Do not stop taking medication without checking with the doctor or nurse practitioner 　C. If side effects of medication occur, call the physician or nurse practitioner so that it may be determined if it needs to be adjusted VII. The patient demonstrates use of home equipment. VIII. The patient states follow-up: 　A. Date of next appointment: _____ 　B. Phone numbers of physician, nurse practitioner, and emergency room: 　　Physician #:_____ 　　Nurse practitioner #:_____ 　　Emergency room #: _____			
Evaluation If patient or significant others are unable to complete some or all of this teaching plan, document evaluation in progress notes.			

	Content/ Reinforcement Delivered Date & RN	Learner Objectives Met Date & RN	Not Applicable

MYOCARDIAL INFARCTION

Purpose

To assist the patient and family in understanding the pathophysiology of coronary artery disease leading to a myocardial infarction.
To assist the patient and family in identifying guidelines for home care related to myocardial infarction.

Content

   I. Anatomy and physiology of the heart muscle
  II. Anatomy and physiology of the heart's blood supply
 III. Atherosclerosis in the development of coronary artery disease
 IV. Objectives of angina teaching plan
  V. Myocardial infarction
    A. Definition
    B. Symptoms
 VI. Risk factors related to individual life style
    A. Controllable
    B. Uncontrollable
    C. Patient's risk factors
VII. Home care of the myocardial infarction patient
    A. Activity
    B. Medications
    C. Diet
    D. Reasons to call physician
    E. Follow-up

Learner Objectives

   I. The patient describes the anatomy and physiology of the heart as a strong hollow muscle that pumps blood to all parts of the body and lungs.
  II. The patient describes the anatomy and physiology of the heart's blood vessels.
    A. Vessels that surround the heart to feed blood containing oxygen to the heart muscle are called *coronary arteries*.
    B. The coronary artery system has three major branches: the right main and circumflex coronary artery supplying blood to both the right and left side of the heart and the left coronary artery supplying blood to the left side of the heart.

	Content/ Reinforcement Delivered Date & RN	Learner Objectives Met Date & RN	Not Applicable

III. The patient describes the development of coronary artery disease from atherosclerosis.
  A. Fatty layers (plaque) form and accumulate on the lining of the coronary arteries.
  B. This plaque is usually made up of cholesterol, which can block the blood vessels and prevent them from delivering blood to the heart muscle.
IV. The patient meets the learner objectives of the angina teaching plan.
 V. The patient describes the physiology of myocardial infarction and the symptoms associated with it.
  A. A myocardial infarction is an injury to an area of the heart muscle caused by a blocked coronary artery.
  B. Soon after the myocardial infarction, the heart begins to heal through formation of scar tissue, which strengthens the damaged muscle.
  C. Symptoms of a myocardial infarction vary with each individual. Some of the most common symptoms are
    1. Chest discomfort
    2. Pain
    3. Pressure that may extend to the neck, jaw, or arms
    4. Nausea
    5. Perspiration
    6. Dizziness
    7. Weakness
    8. Apprehension
  D. Description of the patient's own symptoms: _____
VI. The patient describes a risk factor and states the controllable and uncontrollable risk factors of own life style. Risk factors are certain habits or characteristics that increase a person's chances of developing narrowing of the coronary arteries.
  A. Controllable factors
    1. Smoking
    2. High blood pressure
    3. Increased amounts of fatty substances (cholesterol) in the blood
    4. Stress or tension
    5. Lack of exercise
    6. Obesity
  B. Uncontrollable factors
    1. Diabetes
    2. Family history of coronary artery disease
    3. Males and people over the age of 50
  C. Patient's risk factors
    Controllable
 	
    _____
    _____
    _____			

	Content/ Reinforcement Delivered Date & RN	Learner Objectives Met Date & RN	Not Applicable
Uncontrollable _____ _____ _____			

VII. The patient describes the guidelines for home care during the first 2 weeks after discharge as discussed with the primary nurse and physician:
A. Activity
  1. Walking
   _____
  2. Stairs
   _____
  3. Bathing
   _____
  4. Riding in a car or driving
   _____
  5. Housework
   _____
  6. Sexual activities
   _____
B. Medications. The patient completes the general medication teaching plan.
C. Diet. The patient describes diet restrictions as discussed with dietitian.
  _____
D. Reasons to call the physician
  1. Recurrence of symptoms that brought the patient to the hospital initially
  2. Side effects of medications taken at home
  3. Questions related to activities discussed in the hospital
E. Follow-up
  1. Next appointment: _____
  2. Phone numbers
   Physician: _____
   Emergency room: _____
   Clinic: _____			

The patient or significant others complete the following teaching plans:
  Angina
  Hypertension
  Congestive heart failure
  Cardiac catheterization			

Evaluation			
If patient or significant others are unable to complete some or all of this teaching plan, document evaluation in progress notes.			

GUIDELINES: HOME CARE FOR MYOCARDIAL INFARCTION PATIENT

To the nurse: When designing an activity home care guide for your patient, please use the following information as a reference. You must discuss with the physician involved in the patient's care what this individual patient requires as a proper guide for activity. Plan together using what the patient states as normal routine at home before this hospitalization. Remember that each patient is an individual and the activity guide must be realistic to the person's life style.

Learner Objective VII

The patient describes the activity and diet guidelines for the first 2 weeks after discharge.
A. Walking. When walking at home, stay on level ground or the floor. Do not hurry. Go outside if the weather is mild. If the weather is too cold or too hot, it may cause your heart to work harder.
B. Stairs. When climbing stairs, go up slowly, stopping on each step to rest.
C. Bathing. When showering, avoid hot or very cold water, hurrying, or excessive scrubbing or drying off.
D. Travel in a car. A family member may drive you to a level place for taking your short walks. You can usually take short trips (for example, to the grocery store). When carrying objects, they should weigh less than 5 pounds.
E. Housework. Light housework (for example, help prepare meals or wash dishes), remembering to keep arms at waist level.
F. Sexual activity. Sexual relations with your usual partner requires about the same energy to climb two flights of stairs. Many people participate in sex a month after their heart attack. Give yourselves plenty of time for sex and minimize the chances for interruptions by taking the phone off the hook, making sure that children are occupied.

   If you are tired or have recently eaten a large meal, have sex later.

   Be in a good mood.

   Return to the usual sexual positions unless you would just like to change or these positions seem strenuous to you.

   If you are prone to having angina, take a nitroglycerin before sex. If angina develops during intercourse, stop and rest.

PATIENT HANDOUT FOR HOME CARE

The patient describes the guidelines for home care during the first two weeks after discharge as discussed with the primary nurse and physician.

A. Activity

_____

_____

1. Walking

_____

_____

2. Stairs

_____

_____

3. Bathing

_____

_____

4. Travel in a car

_____

_____

5. Housework

_____

_____

6. Sexual activities

_____

_____

B. Diet restrictions (after discussion with dietitian)

_____

_____

C. Reasons to call the physician
   1. Recurrence of symptoms
   2. Side effects of medication
   3. Questions related to these activities

	Content/ Reinforcement Delivered Date & RN	Learner Objectives Met Date & RN	Not Applicable

PACEMAKER

Purpose

To increase the patient's knowledge of the symptoms, etiology, and treatment of pacemaker-responsive heart disease.
To alleviate the patient's anxiety regarding pacemaker insertion.
To ensure the patient's understanding of pacemaker function.
To assist the patient to live safely with a permanent pacemaker.

Content

    I. Normal anatomy and physiology of the heart
    II. Electrophysiology of the heart
    III. Pathophysiology of the conduction system
    IV. Symptoms due to abnormalities of the conduction system
    V. Components of a permanent pacemaker system
    VI. Functions of an implantable pacemaker
    VII. Preparation for insertion
    VIII. Measurement of the patient's pulse
    IX. Signs and symptoms of pacemaker failure
    X. Use of the transtelephonic home monitor for suspected pacemaker malfunction
    XI. Follow-up

Learner Objectives

    I. The patient describes the normal anatomy and physiology of the heart.
        A. The main function of the heart is to deliver oxygen and nutrients to all of the body's cells.
        B. The heart is a muscular organ consisting of four chambers. The two upper chambers (atria) collect blood, and the lower chambers (ventricles) pump blood to the lungs and throughout the body.
    II. The patient describes the electrical system of the heart.
        A. The main purpose of the electrical system of the heart is to initiate an impulse that can travel along the heart pathways to cause a heartbeat.
        B. The heart has a natural pacemaker (the sinoatrial node) located in the upper portion of the heart. Every pumping action or pulse is preceded by an electrical event starting at the sinoatrial node.
    III. The patient describes the specific etiology of the disease.
        A. Sick sinus syndrome and arrhythmias. Sometimes the natural pacemaker may fail to work and the heart may beat too slowly, too fast, or irregularly. Such changes can reduce the blood and oxygen supply to the body.

	Content/ Reinforcement Delivered Date & RN	Learner Objectives Met Date & RN	Not Applicable
B. Heart block. A blockage somewhere in the electrical pathways causes abnormal conduction and abnormal pumping. A sufficient supply of oxygen and nutrients may not be received from the abnormal heartbeat.			
IV. The patient describes symptoms of a lowered heart rate:			
A. Dizziness			
B. Weakness			
C. Fatigue			
D. Shortness of breath			
E. Chest pain with even slight exertion			
V. The patient describes the components of a pacemaker system.			
A. A pulse generator houses the battery.			
B. A lead carries the energy to the heart.			
VI. The patient describes the function of the pacemaker.			
A. The main function of the implantable pacemaker is to stimulate the heart to beat at an acceptable rate.			
B. The electrical pulses traveling through the lead stimulate the surrounding heart tissue causing the heart to contract or beat.			
C. The electrical pulses of the pacemaker are sent out only when a missed beat is detected. This allows the heart to work on its own, and the pacemaker is used only when needed.			
D. The pacemaker can be programmed (i.e., rate set) depending on the patient's needs.			
VII. The patient describes the preparation for a permanent pacemaker insertion.			
A. An intravenous infusion is started to give access for antibiotic administration before pacemaker insertion.			
B. The procedure usually takes 2 to 2½ hours. Local anesthesia (Xylocaine) is used to numb the area where the doctors work. The patient is awake during the procedure, and the pacemaker can be seen before implantation.			
VIII. The patient describes the pulse relative to the pacemaker.			
A. Every contraction of the heart either from the implantable or natural pacemaker is equal to the pulse felt at the wrist.			
B. To take the pulse, place 2 fingers of one hand on the opposite wrist. Do not press too hard, just enough to feel the steady beat under the skin. Count the beat for 1 minute, using a clock or watch with a sweep second hand.			
IX. The patient describes the signs and symptoms of pacemaker failure.			
A. A recurrence of the symptoms experienced before pacemaker insertion (e.g., dizziness, weakness, short-			

	Content/ Reinforcement Delivered Date & RN	Learner Objectives Met Date & RN	Not Applicable

ness of breath, chest pain) could indicate pacemaker failure.
B. A pulse rate below the set rate of the implantable pacemaker is often a warning that the battery of the pacemaker is getting weak and replacement might be indicated.
X. The patient describes action to be taken if signs of pacemaker failure recur.
  A. With the transtelephonic monitor periodically (usually monthly), pacemaker function may be checked. If pacemaker failure is suspected, call 1-800-223-0500.
  B. Contact the physician or nurse if any signs of pacemaker failure occur.
    Physician #: _____
    Nurse #: _____
XI. The patient describes changes in activities of daily life and follow-up procedure.
  A. There are no specific activity limitations for patients with permanent pacemakers.
  B. Built-in features in the pacemaker protect it from interference produced by electrical devices.
  C. The doctor will discuss any special limitations.
  D. The pacemaker battery usually lasts 6 to 7 years.
  E. An appointment will be scheduled with the doctor in the pacemaker clinic to have staples removed 10 to 12 days after insertion.
    Appointment date: _____
    Physician: _____			

Evaluation If patient or significant others are unable to complete some or all of this teaching plan, document evaluation in progress notes.			

Part II

The Endocrine System

	Content/ Reinforcement Delivered Date & RN	Learner Objectives Met Date & RN	Not Applicable

FOOT CARE FOR THE DIABETIC

Purpose

To provide information to the diabetic patient about good care of the feet.

To prevent complications, i.e., chronic infection and osteomyelitis, requiring prolonged hospital care and possible loss of a limb.

Content

    I. Definition and procedure for foot hygiene
   II. Don'ts of foot care for the diabetic
  III. Care of toenails
  IV. Proper shoes and socks
   V. Reasons to contact physician
  VI. How to contact physician
 VII. Handouts

Learner Objectives

    I. The patient describes the procedure of regular foot care.
      A. Wash feet in warm water and mild soap.
      B. Use soft brush on nails and bottom of feet.
      C. Dry carefully, especially between toes by blotting, not rubbing.
      D. If skin shows signs of dryness, apply pure lanolin ointment immediately after bathing or soaking the feet.
      E. Areas of low sensation or insensitivity occur in diabetic neuropathy, and consequently the "feel of the feet" should not be trusted.
      F. The feet should be inspected carefully in good light once a day. White or pale areas, blisters, or red areas should be called to the attention of the physician.
   II. The patient describes the don'ts of diabetic foot care.
      A. Do not sit with legs crossed.
      B. Never use hot-water bottles or heating pads to warm the feet.
      C. Avoid exposure of the feet to high or low temperatures.
      D. Avoid working areas where there is a possibility of foot injury.
      E. Use caution in placing feet on or near heating registers, care heaters, heat lamps, etc.
      F. Avoid exposure of feet to sun.
  III. The patient describes the proper cutting of toenails and emergency home care of corns and calluses.
      A. File nails using a coarse file with a blunt tip or an emory board. File from the top down, not crosswise as on the fingers.

	Content/ Reinforcement Delivered Date & RN	Learner Objectives Met Date & RN	Not Applicable

B. Cut nails straight across, never curved.
C. Never cut corns or calluses with razor blades or scissors.
D. Do not use corn remedies, corn pads, or adhesive plaster.
E. Do not use strong antiseptics such as iodine, mercury, or phenol.
IV. The patient describes five check points regarding proper fitting shoes and socks:
  A. Proper shoes
    1. Shoes should be made of leather.
    2. Shoes should be roomy across ball of foot.
    3. Shoes should always be lined with a good quality cloth (cotton preferred).
    4. Shoes should have hard toes to safeguard against stubbing.
    5. Shoes should have a soft, pliable upper portion.
  B. Proper socks
    1. White socks should be worn.
    2. Socks should be changed daily and be warm and dry.
    3. Elastic garters should never be worn.
    4. Darns and holes should be avoided since they may lead to blisters.
    5. Socks should be heavy, good quality soft cotton, cotton and wool, or all wool.
V. Patient states skin problems that necessitate a call to the physician:
  A. Redness, swelling, heat, or pain in the feet
  B. Any pus or abnormal drainage from the feet
  C. Ingrown toenail
  D. Any trauma to the feet
VI. Patient states how to contact the physician:
  A. Diabetes clinic #: _____
  B. Emergency room #: _____
VII. Patient takes home handout material.
 	
Evaluation
 	
If patient or significant others are unable to complete some or all of this teaching plan, document evaluation in progress notes.			

	Content/ Reinforcement Delivered Date & RN	Learner Objectives Met Date & RN	Not Applicable

GENERAL ADULT DIABETIC

Purpose

To provide knowledge to the diabetic patient and significant others concerning the etiology, existence, and predominance of diabetes among the adult population.
To provide a knowledge base that will facilitate better diabetes control by the patient.

Content

  I. A basic description of diabetes
 II. Description of the predisposing factors as well as familial and genetic influences of diabetes
III. Review of signs and symptoms common to adult diabetic patients
 IV. A list and explanation of major complications related to diabetes
  V. Discussion of health maintenance
 VI. Discussion of the importance of identification of the patient as a diabetic

Learner Objectives

  I. The patient names the disease and describes its cause. The cause of diabetes mellitus is unknown, but it is characterized by an elevation of blood sugar secondary to the inability of the pancreas to produce sufficient insulin.
 II. The patient states the influence of predisposing factors, family health history, and own diabetes:
      A. Obesity
      B. Lack of exercise
      C. Coronary artery disease
      D. Hypertension
III. The patient names the signs and symptoms of diabetes:
      A. Frequent urination
      B. Excessive thirst
      C. Headache
      D. Weakness
      E. Fatigue
      F. Dizziness
      G. Dry, hot skin
      H. Nausea, vomiting
      I. Abdominal cramps
 IV. The patient states the complications of diabetes:
      A. Loss of eyesight
      B. Kidney failure

	Content/ Reinforcement Delivered Date & RN	Learner Objectives Met Date & RN	Not Applicable

C. Frequent infection
D. Foot ulcers
E. Heart attack
V. The patient states the health interventions necessary to prevent or allay these complications:
  A. Routine checkups with physician
  B. Sufficient knowledge of insulin
  C. Sufficient knowledge of proper nutrition
  D. Proper knowledge regarding contact numbers with physician or emergency room if in trouble
VI. Patient states the importance of wearing a medic alert bracelet or medical identification.
  A. In case of bizarre behavior the patient will be easily identified as having diabetes and needing treatment (glucose).
  B. If in an accident, glucose would not be given inadvertently.
  C. If found in a coma, the patient would be brought to the hospital immediately.			

Evaluation If patient or significant others are unable to complete some or all of this teaching plan, document evaluation in progress notes.			

	Content/ Reinforcement Delivered Date & RN	Learner Objectives Met Date & RN	Not Applicable

HYPO- AND HYPERGLYCEMIA

Purpose

To educate the diabetic patient about the signs and symptoms of insulin reaction and diabetic ketoacidosis.
To help the patient prevent these symptoms and to take proper action if they occur.

Content

I. Signs and symptoms of hypoglycemia
II. Reasons for hypoglycemia and preventative measures
III. Proper course of action for hypoglycemia
IV. Signs and symptoms of hyperglycemia
V. Reason for hyperglycemia and preventative measures
VI. Proper course of action for hyperglycemia
VII. How to contact the physician

Learner Objectives

I. The patient describes signs and symptoms of hypoglycemia (low blood sugar):
    1. Fatigue
    2. Headache
    3. Drowsiness
    4. Tremors
    5. Weakness
    6. Sweating
    7. Negative urine sugar test
    All of these symptoms occur over a short period.
II. The patient describes the reasons for hypoglycemia and preventative measures:
A. Reasons
    1. Failure to eat enough food when taking insulin
    2. Excessive exercise
    3. Excessive insulin dose
    4. Result of illness such as nausea, vomiting, or diarrhea
B. Preventative measures
    1. Never skip a meal when on insulin.
    2. Increase caloric intake if vigorous exercise is anticipated.
    3. Always carry hard candy in form of Life Savers (approximately 10 gm) in a pocket.
    4. Pay careful attention to drawing up and administering the correct dose of insulin every day.
    5. Maintain adequate liquid carbohydrate intake.

	Content/ Reinforcement Delivered Date & RN	Learner Objectives Met Date & RN	Not Applicable
6. Medic-alert bracelet or some form of identification should be carried at all times by diabetic patients in case of collapse.			
III. The patient describes the proper action or intervention for hypoglycemia.			
A. Eat some form of concentrated sugar such as Life Savers or sugar cubes if not at home.			
B. If at home, drink orange juice or any liquid containing sugar.			
C. If symptoms persist, test urine sugar and call the physician.			
D. The patient should be brought to the emergency room if these actions are not effective.			
IV. The patient describes the signs and symptoms of hyperglycemia (high blood sugar):			
A. Frequent urination			
B. Excessive thirst			
C. Headache			
D. Weakness			
E. Fatigue			
F. Dizziness			
G. Dry, hot flushed skin			
H. Nausea			
I. Vomiting			
J. Abdominal cramps			
K. Urine glucose at 4+ and ketones present			
These symptoms will have a slow, gradual onset.			
V. The patient describes the reasons for hyperglycemia and preventative measures:			
A. Reasons			
1. Increase in carbohydrate intake for morning insulin			
2. Omission of insulin			
3. Infection			
4. Illness			
5. Emotional stress			
B. Preventative measures			
1. Avoid overeating; follow diet			
2. Check insulin dosage carefully			
3. Exercise sufficiently			
4. Check urine regularly			
5. Medic-alert bracelet or some form of identification should be carried at all times in case of collapse			
6. Visit physician regularly			
VI. The patient describes proper action or intervention for hyperglycemia.			
A. If 4+ glycosuria is present or symptoms of hyperglycemia are present, contact physician or go to an emergency room *immediately*.			

	Content/ Reinforcement Delivered Date & RN	Learner Objectives Met Date & RN	Not Applicable
B. If ketones in urine are present, notify physician or go to an emergency room *immediately*.			
VII. The patient states how to contact doctor and the emergency room:			
A. Physician #: _____			
B. Emergency room #: _____			

Evaluation

If patient or significant others are unable to complete some or all of this teaching plan, document evaluation in progress notes.

	Content/ Reinforcement Delivered	Learner Objectives Met	Not Applicable
	Date & RN	Date & RN	

INSULIN INJECTION

Purpose

To enable the insulin-dependent diabetic patient to administer insulin properly.
To increase the insulin-dependent diabetic patient's knowledge about the medical regimen.

Content

I. Description of the types of insulin as they relate to
   A. Dosage and concentration
   B. Onset, peak, and duration of action
   C. Special dietary precautions
   D. Storage
II. Demonstration of the techniques used to draw up insulin
III. Supervision of return demonstration
IV. Handouts

Learner Objectives

(The patient meets the objectives of the general diabetes and hypo- and hyperglycemia teaching plan.)
I. The patient names the insulin and describes the medication as it relates to
   A. Type of insulin: _____
      Dosage: _____units
      Strength: _____
   B. Common types of insulin
     1. NPH
       a) Onset of action: ½ hour after injection
       b) Peak of action: 8 hours after injection
       c) Duration of action: 18 to 22 hours after injection
     2. Lente
       a) Onset of action: 1 to 2 hours after injection
       b) Peak of action: 10 to 16 hours after injection
       c) Duration of action: 18 to 30 hours after injection
     3. Regular (Chrystalline)
       a) Onset of action: ½ hour after injection
       b) Peak of action: 2 to 4 hours after injection
       c) Duration of action: 6 to 8 hours after injection
   C. Special dietary precautions
     1. Usually 1,500 calories or 1,800 calories, ADA, 60% carbohydrate, 20% fat, and 20% protein.
     2. Individual dietary instruction handout material.

	Content/ Reinforcement Delivered Date & RN	Learner Objectives Met Date & RN	Not Applicable

D. Storage. Insulin is preferably stored in the refrigerator. It can also be kept in a cool, dark place away from heat or sunlight.
II. The patient demonstrates the proper insulin injection techniques by
  A. Explaining the reason for rotating the site of injection and describing how to choose these sites.
    1. Injection into the same site will cause poor absorption due to swelling and weakness of the subcutaneous fat.
    2. The choice of sites includes:
      a) Right and left deltoid area
      b) Right and left anterior thigh
      c) Whole area of abdominal fat
      d) Different site every day in a clockwise direction
  B. Properly administering own insulin
    1. Wash hands.
    2. Rotate the insulin bottle.
    3. Wash the rubber top of the bottle with alcohol.
    4. Inject air into the bottle.
    5. Turn the bottle upside down.
    6. Pull the plunger back to the appropriate dose.
    7. Wash the area of skin with alcohol.
    8. Hold the skin taut.
    9. Puncture the skin, pushing the needle all the way down at a 90° angle.
    10. Aspirate slightly to check for blood.
    11. Inject the insulin.
    12. Pull the needle out quickly.
III. Using this technique, the patient demonstrates three times the ability to draw up correctly various doses of insulin according to sterile technique.
IV. The patient takes handouts and educational materials home and states where to find information on the particular type of insulin.			

Evaluation

If patient or significant others are unable to complete some or all of this teaching plan, document evaluation in progress notes.

	Content/ Reinforcement Delivered Date & RN	Learner Objectives Met Date & RN	Not Applicable

URINE TESTING FOR THE DIABETIC

Purpose

To provide the diabetic patient with knowledge of the technique and understanding of the purpose of testing urine for glucose and acetone.
To provide the diabetic patient with the means to measure and record the results of urine glucose tests.

Content

    I. Explanation of why urine is tested
   II. Explanation of how often and when to test urine
  III. Demonstration of the principles involved in testing by the appropriate method
  IV. Principles involved in recording results of test
   V. Important precautions to ensure accurate test results
  VI. Reasons to notify physician
 VII. How to contact physician
VIII. Review hypoglycemia and hyperglycemia teaching plan

Learner Objectives

   I. The patient explains why urine is tested.
     A. It gives a picture of how the body is handling its internal supply of sugar.
     B. It is a monitor to determine if a sufficient amount of insulin is being taken daily to control the blood sugar level.
     C. It determines whether diet, medication, and exercise are in balance at all times.
     D. It is used as an indication of illness.
  II. The patient describes the basic principles of how often and when to test.
     A. The basic principles of each procedure are covered in learner objective III.
     B. Urine should be checked three to four times daily:
       1. A double void specimen in the morning
       2. One half-hour before lunch
       3. One half-hour before dinner
       4. At bedtime
     C. Urine testing is especially important during pregnancy or illness.
 III. The patient demonstrates the principles of testing urine by the appropriate method. The patient
     A. Observes the nurse doing the procedure.

	Content/ Reinforcement Delivered Date & RN	Learner Objectives Met Date & RN	Not Applicable

B. Demonstrates accurately the correct procedure for testing the urine for sugar and acetone.
  1. Descriptions
    a) Keto-diastix by Ames. Dip stick in urine, wait 15 seconds for ketones, wait 30 seconds for glucose, compare to chart on bottles, record in percentage of glucose.
    b) Diastix by Ames. One square measures glucose in 30 seconds; dip stick method, compare to chart on bottle.
    c) Test-tape by Lilly. Least expensive, least accurate. Dip stick method; wait 1 full minute after dipping stick in urine; compare to chart on bottle.
    d) Clinitest method. Most accurate, time-consuming, and awkward for the businessman, school-age diabetic, and people away from home.
  2. Procedures
    a) Five-drop Clinitest method
      (1) Place 5 drops of urine in a test tube.
      (2) Add 10 drops of water.
      (3) Add 1 Clinitest tablet.
      (4) Await reaction.
      (5) Compare tablet color to the chart on the bottle.
    b) Two-drop Clinitest method
      (1) Place 2 drops of urine in a test tube.
      (2) Add 10 drops of water.
      (3) Add 1 Clinitest tablet.
      (4) Await reaction.
      (5) A special 2-drop QTT method chart is needed for comparison. This method is used if glucose in the urine is greater than 2%. This method will measure a glucose concentration of up to 5%.
      (6) Test for acetone.
    c) Ketostix by Ames
      (1) Dip stick in urine.
      (2) Wait 15 seconds.
      (3) Compare tablet color to the chart on the bottle.
    d) Acetest tablet
      (1) Place 1 drop of urine on the tablet.
      (2) Wait 30 seconds.
      (3) Compare tablet color to the chart on the bottle.
C. The patient takes the initiative to do the procedure.			

	Content/ Reinforcement Delivered	Learner Objectives Met	Not Applicable
	Date & RN	Date & RN	

IV. The patient accurately states the principles involved in recording the test results in a book and describes the importance of keeping a record.
  A. The patient records accurately the results obtained from appropriate urine-testing method under proper date, time indicating any unusual occurrence, e.g., overeating, stress, excessive exercise.
  B. A record is important to indicate over a period of time how the body is using its glucose and to determine if not enough or too much insulin is being taken daily.
V. The patient states important precautions for accurate test results.
  A. Keep all bottles in a cool dark place.
  B. Keep bottles tightly covered. After opening bottles, replace caps immediately.
  C. Keep Clinitest tablets away from sunlight and direct heat.
  D. Never use sticks or tablets that have changed color.
  E. Handle carefully and store safely away from oral medications and out of the reach of children.
  F. Be sure that the color chart matches the method of urine testing being done.
VI. The patient states reasons to notify the physician:
  A. Urine glucose exceeding
  _____
  (percentage to be determined by physician)
  B. Presence of ketones in the urine
  C. Illness or infection
  D. Vomiting or diarrhea
  E. Frequent negative urines
  F. Symptoms of hypoglycemia (see hypoglycemia and hyperglycemia teaching plan)
VII. The patient states how to contact the physician:
Diabetes clinic # _____
VIII. The patient meets the objectives of the hypoglycemia and hyperglycemia teaching plan.
 	
Evaluation
 	
If patient or significant others are unable to complete some or all of this teaching plan, document evaluation in progress notes.			

Part III

The Gastrointestinal System

	Content/ Reinforcement Delivered Date & RN	Learner Objectives Met Date & RN	Not Applicable

CHOLECYSTECTOMY

Purpose

To educate the patient about the basic function of the gallbladder and about gallbladder disease.
To decrease the patient's level of anxiety about preoperative and postoperative expectations and to increase the patient's compliance with medical and nursing intervention.

Content

    I. Function of the gallbladder
   II. Brief overview of gallbladder disease
  III. Need for surgical repair
  IV. Preoperative routines
   V. Postoperative routines
  VI. Discharge planning
 VII. Reasons to contact the physician
VIII. Follow-up

Learner Objectives

   I. The patient verbalizes an understanding of the function of the gallbladder.
     A. The gallbladder is located on the undersurface of the liver, which is located in the right upper quadrant of the abdomen.
     B. The main function of the gallbladder is to concentrate and store bile, which enters it by way of the liver.
     C. Digestion stimulates the gallbladder, which ejects concentrated bile into the duodenum (the first portion of the small intestine), where it helps in the digestion of fats.
  II. The patient states basic information regarding gallbladder disease.
     A. Cholelithiasis is the medical term for gallstones.
        1. Gallstones are formed from solid particles.
        2. Gallstones vary in size, shape, and consistency.
     B. Cholecystitis is an inflammation of the gallbladder most frequently caused by infection.
     C. Symptoms of gallbladder disease include
        1. Fullness and belching after meals.
        2. Heartburn and chronic pain in the upper right abdomen.
        3. Excruciating upper right abdominal pain (radiates to back or right shoulder) associated with nausea and vomiting.

	Content/ Reinforcement Delivered Date & RN	Learner Objectives Met Date & RN	Not Applicable

4. An onset of symptoms several hours after eating fried or fatty foods. Nausea may occur because of an inability of the body to digest fats.
 	
III. The patient states the need for surgical intervention.
  A. Cholecystectomy is the removal of the gallbladder.
  B. Surgical intervention is necessary for longstanding symptoms of gallbladder disease.
 	
IV. The patient states the preoperative routine:
  A. The following diagnostic tests are completed
    1. Blood tests
    2. Urine samples
    3. Chest x-ray
    4. Electrocardiogram
    5. Oral cholecystogram
    6. Intravenous cholangiogram
  B. An informed consent or signed operative permit is obtained after the doctor has explained the procedure to the patient.
  C. Skin preparation consists of a scrub to the preoperative area with antiseptic soap the night before surgery.
  D. Nothing by mouth is allowed after midnight the night before surgery.
  E. Preoperative medications are given just before leaving the floor to induce relaxation and sleepiness.
  F. Intravenous therapy is given to maintain fluid balance throughout surgery and the postoperative period.
  G. An anesthesiologist discusses the options and assists in the decision of what anesthesia will be used.
 	
V. The patient states the postoperative routine.
  A. The patient wakens in the recovery room.
  B. Intravenous therapy continues for several days until the patient is tolerating a diet.
  C. There is a large dressing over the right upper abdomen. A drain may also be placed in this area. The drain may be one of three types: a trans-hepatic tube (T-tube), a penrose drain, or a Jackson-Pratt drain.
    1. A T-tube is placed in the gallbladder duct to allow bile to drain to the outside into a plastic bag. This gives the ducts the opportunity to heal. The T-tube is usually removed 1 to 2 days before discharge.
    2. A penrose drain or a Jackson-Pratt drain is placed into the space left in the body after the gallbladder is removed. This area tends to collect fluid immediately after surgery and needs to be drained.			

	Content/ Reinforcement Delivered Date & RN	Learner Objectives Met Date & RN	Not Applicable

D. A nasogastric tube is placed after anesthesia to relieve distention of the stomach and gastrointestinal tract.
   1. The nasogastric tube remains in place until gas is passed rectally and bowel sounds can be heard with a stethoscope, usually 1 to 3 days.
   2. While the nasogastric tube is in place, the patient may not eat or drink.
E. Respiratory treatments are necessary to mobilize lung secretions caused by decreased mobility and shallow breathing.
   1. Because the incision for the cholecystectomy is under the right rib cage, an attempt is made to splint the incision by unconsciously taking shallow breaths.
   2. Coughing, deep breathing, and ambulation help to loosen secretions and expand the airways.
F. Activity may initially be uncomfortable for the patient. It may be necessary to take pain medication before ambulation or other activity.
G. The diet will be advanced slowly after the nasogastric tube is taken out. Fatty foods must be avoided, but otherwise a normal diet may be resumed.
 	
VI. The patient states instructions regarding discharge.
A. Do not return to work or drive until further instruction is received at the first clinic appointment.
B. Care of the suture line follows:
   1. No dressing or staples are left at the time of discharge.
   2. If steri-strips are in place, a shower may be taken. Pat dry, do not rub the strip; they will fall off by themselves.
   3. The suture line should be inspected daily for signs of redness, swelling, or drainage.
C. The patient meets the objective of the medication teaching plan for all discharge medication.
 	
VII. The patient states reasons to contact the doctor:
A. Any change in the suture line:
   1. Redness
   2. Swelling
   3. Drainage
B. Increased pain
C. Temperature over 99°F
D. Shaking, chills
 	
VIII. The patient states follow-up care:
A. Follow-up appointment: _____			

	Content/ Reinforcement Delivered Date & RN	Learner Objectives Met Date & RN	Not Applicable
B. Date: _____ C. Physician phone number: _____			
Evaluation If patient or significant others are unable to complete some or all of this teaching plan, document evaluation in progress notes.			

	Content/ Reinforcement Delivered Date & RN	Learner Objectives Met Date & RN	Not Applicable
CONSTIPATION **Purpose** To make the patient aware that constipation is a common problem but may also be a sign of serious disease. To provide patient with information needed to treat and prevent constipation. **Content** I. Definition of constipation in relation to normal bowel habits II. Common causes and symptoms of constipation III. Treatment of the constipated patient IV. Patient handout			
Learner Objectives I. The patient defines constipation in terms of frequency and symptomatology.			
II. Patient identifies causes of constipation.			
III. Patient describes the methods that will be used to prevent constipation.			
IV. Patient takes home constipation handout.			
Evaluation If patient or significant others are unable to complete some or all of this teaching plan, document evaluation in progress notes.			

GUIDELINES: CONSTIPATION

Treatment of constipation is directed toward the underlying disorder. To determine the cause, the nurse must fully evaluate the learning needs and establish a teaching regimen. The following is an example of an evaluation tool.

Evaluation of the Constipated Patient

Name _____

History (Background information can be drawn from front sheet of assessment.)

Married [   ]   Single [   ]   Divorced [   ]
    Children: [   ] Yes   [   ] No
Nationality _____
Social history _____
Alcohol [   ] How much _____
Smoke [   ] How much _____
Occupation _____
Recent travel _____
Weight gain [   ]   Weight loss [   ] _____
Food likes (List 5 most frequently eaten foods.)
1. _____
2. _____
3. _____
4. _____
5. _____
Food dislikes (List 5 most disliked foods.)
1. _____
2. _____
3. _____
4. _____
5. _____
Food intolerances and allergies _____

_____
Meals per day _____
Snacks per day _____
NURSING ASSESSMENT
General physical appearance
In pain [   ] Yes   [   ] No
Skin turgor _____

Skin color _____
Hair distribution _____
General state of hydration _____
Jaundice _____
Halitosis _____
Usual bowel habits (Allow the patient to state in own words what is normal.)
Movements per day _____
Movements per week (if not daily) _____
Timing of movements _____
Consistency

Varies [ ]	Normal size [ ]
Hard [ ]	Straining on defecation [ ]
Soft [ ]	Mucus [ ]
Pebblelike [ ]	Food particles [ ]
Blood [ ]	

Use of laxatives   [   ] Yes [   ] No
                      What kind/how often? _____
Use of antacids   [   ] Yes [   ] No
                      What kind/how often? _____
Taking medication   [   ] Yes [   ] No
                      Which ones? _____
Usual sleep pattern
    Up at night [   ]   To bed late [   ]
    Restless [   ]   Up early [   ]
Pathophysiology

Abdominal pain [ ]	Melena [ ]
Referred pain [ ]	Rectal itching [ ]
Obstipation [ ]	Rectal burning [ ]
Flatus [ ]	Color of stool [ ]
Belching [ ]	Hemorrhoids [ ]
Heartburn [ ]	Recent changes in bowel habits [ ]
Anorexia [ ]	Ascites/bloating [ ]
Nausea [ ]	Tenesmus [ ]
Vomiting [ ]	Nocturnal diarrhea [ ]
Hematemesis [ ]	Fever/flushing [ ]
History of ulcer [ ]	Tachycardia [ ]
Vascular disease [ ]	Ischemia of colon [ ]

Attitude toward work _____
Pressures at home _____
Interpersonal difficulty _____

PATIENT HANDOUT: INFORMATION ON CONSTIPATION

What is constipation? Constipation is a sluggish action of the bowel. It is usually accompanied by prolonged passing of hard stools, decreased number of bowel movements, or small pebblelike stools. Often you may experience low back pain, fatigue, headaches, or a feeling of fullness.

What causes constipation? Constipation is a common problem but can be a warning of more serious disease. If prolonged constipation is a change from your normal bowel habits or blood can be seen in your bowel movements, medical advice should be sought. Simple everyday constipation is usually the result of one of the following:

1. Poor dietary habits. Persons with low fiber intake, low total food intake, and low fluid intake will have fewer stools.
2. Lack of activity. When at rest or in a recumbent position, the usual motion of the bowel is lessened. Decreased activity may be associated with illness, age, or a change in life style.
3. Environmental influences. Travel, poor bathroom facilities, and unfamiliar surroundings can change your normal bowel routine.
4. Emotions. During periods of emotional stress your bowel habits may change.
5. Ignoring the urge to pass stool. Neglecting your normal bowel habits disturbs the natural process of bowel elimination.
6. Drugs. Medications such as antacids and pain medication and the chronic use of laxatives may decrease the natural motion of the bowel.

How can I help myself?

1. Diet
   a. Begin to include more of the following foods:
      Fruit juices
      Fresh and stewed fruits
      100% bran (make sure that you drink lots of fluid with bran)
      Green leafy vegetables
      At least 10 glasses of fluid daily
   b. Limit the following foods:
      White sugar
      Pastas
      Pastries
2. Activity
   a. Increase your daily activity.
   b. Include mild exercise after meals.
3. Environment. Be aware that many things in your environment can change your normal bowel habits. Anticipate them and plan how you will adjust your diet, activity, and elimination pattern as your daily routine changes.
4. Regulate your bowel habits.
   a. Set a certain time every day that is quiet and uninterrupted.
   b. Do not ignore the urge to empty your bowels.
5. Patience. These changes will not help overnight.

What about laxatives? Unfortunately laxatives are used to treat constipation rather than prevent it. Since laxatives may be habit-forming and harmful to the bowel, it is wiser to prevent constipation. Laxatives should be used regularly only with the advice of a physician.

	Content/ Reinforcement Delivered Date & RN	Learner Objectives Met Date & RN	Not Applicable

DISCHARGE TEACHING FOR POSTOPERATIVE TONSILLECTOMY AND ADENOIDECTOMY PATIENT
 	
Purpose
 	
To decrease parental and child anxiety and ensure parents' ability to safely care for the child at home.
 	
Content
 	
    I. Normal recovery course at home
   II. Activity
  III. Diet
  IV. Mouth care
   V. Reasons to notify the physician
  VI. Follow-up			

Learner Objectives
 	
    I. The parents and child (if the age is appropriate) describe normal recovery at home:
       A. Lethargy. There will be a period of time during which the child is more sleepy than usual. This will resolve in several days.
       B. Pain. It is expected that the child will complain of throat pain usually associated with swallowing. The pain should resolve within several days.
       C. Oozing. Oozing can be described as "old blood," dark brown in color, often mixed with saliva. Sometimes it will be noted on the child's pillow. This is an expected occurrence and should resolve within several days.
   II. The parents and child (if the age is appropriate) describe activity at home.
       A. Strenuous activity should be avoided in order that healing at the surgical site will not be interrupted.
       B. The child does not have to spend the day in bed. However, time should be allotted for resting.
       C. The parents should identify types of nonstrenuous activity that their child enjoys.
  III. The parents and child (if the age is appropriate) state the dietary restrictions necessary to promote the healing process:
       A. General restrictions. Foods that are very hot or very cold can disturb healing. Also to be avoided are foods that are crunchy or sharp, e.g., potato chips.
       B. Full liquids. Full liquids are likely to be the child's diet at discharge. Foods included in this group are custard,			

	Content/ Reinforcement Delivered Date & RN	Learner Objectives Met Date & RN	Not Applicable

ice cream (plain), egg nog, soups (plain). The parents list the following full liquid choices that their child prefers: _____
 C. Soft diet. After 3 to 4 days at home, the child may graduate to a soft diet. Foods included in this group are foods that are literally soft and therefore cannot traumatize healing tissue. Included are foods like cooked vegetables, soft meats (e.g., hamburger), and eggs. The parents list the following soft diet foods that their child prefers.
 IV. The parents and child (if the age is appropriate) describe mouth care.
   A. Many children who have had tonsillectomies have a foul mouth odor.
   B. Gargling is an irritant and should be avoided.
   C. The child should be encouraged to rinse with salt and warm water.
   D. Breath fresheners can be used.
   E. A toothbrush can be used carefully.
   F. As the child begins to eat and drink, the odor should disappear.
 V. The parents and child (if the age is appropriate) state the following reasons to notify the doctor:
   A. Elevated temperature. A temperature greater than _____ for more than 24 hours should be reported to the doctor. This may be a sign of infection.
   B. Mouth odor or oozing. Mouth odor and oozing that persist for more than several days may be a sign of infection and should be reported to the doctor.
   C. Fluids. If a child is refusing to drink or is vomiting persistently, dehydration may occur. This should be reported to the doctor.
   D. Bright red blood. Occasionally persistent coughing or vomiting may reopen the surgical wound. This causes fresh bleeding. This bleeding is different from oozing in that the blood is bright red in color. Before the appearance of blood, the child may become very pale and quiet or the child may feel faint. Any appearance of bright red blood should be reported to the physician immediately. If the child is actively vomiting bright red blood, it should be considered an emergency and the child should be taken immediately to the closest emergency room.
 The doctor's number is _____
 The emergency room phone number is _____
 The emergency room closest to home is _____
 Phone number is _____			

	Content/ Reinforcement Delivered Date & RN	Learner Objectives Met Date & RN	Not Applicable
VI. The parents and child (if the age is appropriate) state the child's follow-up appointment. A. The appointment is on _____ at _____. B. For questions or concerns, call _____ at _____.			
Evaluation If patient or significant others are unable to complete some or all of this teaching plan, document evaluation in progress notes.			

	Content/ Reinforcement Delivered Date & RN	Learner Objectives Met Date & RN	Not Applicable

DUODENAL ULCER

Purpose

To give the patient with a duodenal ulcer an understanding of the disease process and prescribed therapeutic regimen.
To increase awareness of factors that contribute to ulcer disease.

Content

    I. Normal digestive process
    II. Pathophysiology of an ulcer
    III. Common causes of an ulcer
    IV. Signs and symptoms of an ulcer
    V. Treatment of an ulcer and factors that may interfere with treatment
    VI. Potential complications of ulcers
    VII. Reasons to contact physician
    VIII. Follow-up

Learner Objectives

    I. The patient describes the digestive process as a process by which food is broken down and absorbed to provide the body with needed nutrients and other substances.
    II. The patient describes the development of an ulcer as an erosion or hole in the lining of the stomach or duodenum (small intestine).
    III. The patient states the following as causes of an ulcer:
      A. Increased acid production
      B. Irritating substances, e.g., alcohol
      C. Certain medications, e.g., aspirin
      D. Problems with the stomach lining, e.g., poor blood supply
    IV. The patient states at least three of the following as symptoms of an ulcer:
      *A. Burning, aching epigastric pain between meals
      *B. Pain during the night or on arising
      *C. Pain relieved with food, milk, or antacids
      D. Nausea or vomiting
      E. Loss of appetite
      F. Weight loss
    V. A. The patient states the prescribed treatment and its rationale.
        1. The patient meets the objectives of the medication teaching plan for each medication (including antacids).

---
*Must be stated by the patient.

	Content/ Reinforcement Delivered Date & RN	Learner Objectives Met Date & RN	Not Applicable

2. Small, frequent meals are prescribed because the presence of food decreases the acidity of the stomach and duodenum.
3. Avoidance of items in section V, B, is necessary because they are irritating to the stomach lining.
B. The patient states five factors that interfere with the treatment or make ulcers worse:
  1. Coffee, tea, cola
  2. Alcohol
  3. Aspirin
  4. Cigarette smoking
  5. Stress
VI. The patient states potential complications of ulcers and their symptoms:
A. GI bleeding
  1. Passage of bright red blood per rectum
  2. Passage of black tarry stools
  3. Vomiting blood or coffee ground material
  4. Dizziness when standing
  5. Pallor
B. Obstruction
  1. Constipation
  2. Increased abdominal pain
  3. Abdominal fullness or distention
VII. The patient states the reasons to contact the physician:
A. Burning, aching pain between meals or during the night. Pain is relieved by food, milk or antacids.
B. Nausea, vomiting, weight loss, loss of appetite.
C. Bright red blood per rectum, black tarry stools, vomiting blood or coffee ground material, dizziness when standing.
D. Diarrhea, constipation, or abdominal distention.
VIII. The patient states follow-up:
A. Follow-up appointment: _____
B. Telephone numbers
  Physician: _____
  Emergency room: _____		

Evaluation If patient or significant others are unable to complete some or all of this teaching plan, document evaluation in progress notes.		

	Content/ Reinforcement Delivered Date & RN	Learner Objectives Met Date & RN	Not Applicable

GASTROSTOMY: CARE OF THE SITE, APPLICATION OF THE DRESSING, AND FEEDING
 	
Purpose
 	
To familiarize patient and significant others with gastrostomy wound and its proper care.
To teach patient and significant others to accomplish gastrostomy feeding.
 	
Content
 	
  I. Purpose of gastrostomy tube
  II. Description of gastrostomy tube
  III. Gastrostomy care
  IV. Gastrostomy feeding
  V. Care required for dislodged gastrostomy tube
  VI. Items required for gastrostomy care and feeding
  VII. Reasons to contact physician
  VIII. Follow-up
 	
Learner Objectives
 	
  I. The parent and significant others state that the gastrostomy is a temporary (permanent) means of feeding the child when the normal passage of food into the stomach is prevented.
  II. The parent and significant others point to the area of the abdomen where the gastrostomy tube is located and state that:
    A. The tube is a specially tipped latex tube that is passed through several layers of abdominal tissue into the stomach.
    B. The tube is anchored by a mushroom- or bulblike tip without sutures (except in the initial post-op week or so).
    C. The tube is secured by a special dressing that prevents tension on the wound and guards against accidental dislodgement.
  III. The parent and significant others successfully demonstrate cleansing the gastrostomy site and accomplishing a secure dressing.
    A. Dressings are changed every third day and as necessary.
    B. When the dressing is removed, the wound should be examined for
      1. Redness
      2. Swelling
      3. Drainage			

	Content/ Reinforcement Delivered Date & RN	Learner Objectives Met Date & RN	Not Applicable

If any of these signs is seen, the physician should be notified.

C. The site is then washed with warm water and mild soap and dried well.

D. The dressing is then applied and is compact and secure.

IV. The parent and significant others describe and demonstrate the gastrostomy feeding:

  A. Equipment
1. Irrigating syringe
2. Screw clamp
3. Prepared feeding
4. Pacifier as necessary

  B. Feeding procedure
1. Person doing feeding should be seated comfortably with child secure.
2. Unclamp gastrostomy tube.
3. Attach irrigating syringe without plunger (plunger is rarely used, as feeding is added to syringe and height above child's stomach is adjusted to allow feeding to run at 2 to 3 cc/min.).
4. When feeding is finished, tube is flushed with water or air as directed by physician.
5. Child may be "burped" by briefly leaving tube open to air.
6. When feeding is finished, tube is clamped and end covered with dry sponge.
7. Feeding should be held and physician notified if child is distended or is vomiting.

V. Parent and significant others state what to do if tube becomes dislodged.

  A. Cover site with clean bandage, tightly taped.

  B. Bring child to emergency room as quickly as possible to have tube replaced.

  C. Bring displaced tube with child to emergency room.

VI. Parent and significant others list items needed for gastrostomy care and feeding:

  A. Dressing change
1. Four 1-inch wide adhesive strips 3 inches long—2 of these are half-split lengthwise
2. Benzoin and applicator sticks
3. Two 2 × 2 inch gauze folded to be 1 × 1 inch and cut in a Y
4. Warm water

  B. Feeding
1. 60-cc irrigating syringe
2. Measuring cup
3. Feeding mixture

	Content/Reinforcement Delivered Date & RN	Learner Objectives Met Date & RN	Not Applicable

4. Hoffman clamp
5. Elastic and gauze (to cover tube after feeding)
VII. Patient and parents state reasons to contact physician:
 A. _____
 B. _____
 C. _____
 D. _____
VIII. Patient and parents describe follow-up:
 A. Next appointment with
  Physician: _____
 B. Telephone numbers for problems
  Physician: _____
  Emergency room: _____			

Evaluation If patient or significant others are unable to complete some or all of this teaching plan, document evaluation in progress notes.			

GUIDELINES: GASTROSTOMY

Patients and parents should learn to care for the gastrostomy wound and be able to accomplish feeding successfully via the gastrostomy tube. Each should also be able to relate location of tube and demonstrate knowledge of what would happen if tube became dislodged. A knowledge of equipment essential to wound care and feeding is necessary.

I. The patient or significant other describes the purpose and location of the gastrostomy tube.

II. Before attempting to show patient and parents the gastrostomy feeding, an explanation of the tube's purpose and its location might be a good place to start. The dressed wound is often enough to see in the first lesson.

III. The parent or significant other successfully demonstrates cleansing the gastrostomy site and accomplishing a secure dressing.

In the next session, the nurse might encourage the parent to view the wound site and observe the nurse doing the dressing. Dressing changes are done every third day, but may be redone any time for demonstration. After the wound is undressed, the site should be examined for redness, swelling, and drainage. The area around the tube should be cleansed with warm water and dried well. The gastrostomy dressing is applied to protect the site and maintain the tube securely, taut against the stomach wall. A tube that is allowed to slip in and out will cause an erosion and subsequent infection of the site. If dressing adherence has been a problem, apply benzoin to a 1-inch-wide area around the gastrostomy tube. The area should be allowed to dry until it is still somewhat tacky. Fold in half a 2-inch-square gauze bandage

twice so that a 1-inch square remains. Cut the 1-inch square in a Y-shape and place it around the base of the tube (Figure 2A). Fold and cut a second bandage and place it around the base of the tube to provide adequate coverage. Using 1-inch-wide adhesive tape, cut four strips, each 3 inches in length. The first two are used to anchor the gauze bandage to the skin (Figure 2B). Split each of the remaining strips in half lengthwise until the midpoint is reached (Figure 2C). Anchor the nonsplit end of the tape to the skin and gauze surrounding the tube. Then stretch one of the split ends of tape across the dressing and wrap the other around the base of the tube. Use one hand to wrap the tape and the other to pull the gastrostomy tube snug against the abdominal wall (Figure 2D). This keeps the tube from retracting. Place the second split strip over the dressing and tube in the opposite direction. The entire dressing should thus be compact and secure.

IV. The parent or significant other demonstrates the gastrostomy feeding.

Once the parents are familiar with the gastrostomy wound and its purpose, they may undertake the responsibility for feeding the patient and changing the dressing under nursing supervision. Feedings are accomplished by placing a 60-cc irrigating syringe into the gastrostomy tube. The feeding runs in by gravity. The rate of flow for infants should be 2 to 3 cc/minute. The rate may be increased as comfortable for an older child or adult. If the feeding does not run freely, milking the tube toward the patient may help. One should never push the entire feeding using the syringe plunger. Care should be taken to keep the feeding dilute enough to allow free flow. An appar-

---

Figure 2 Bandaging a Gastrostomy

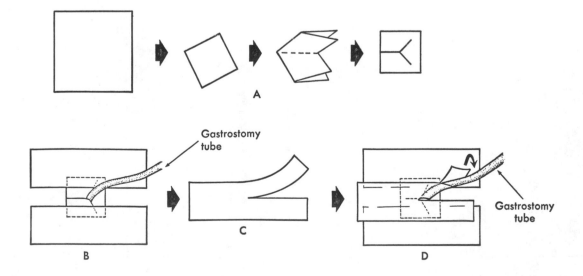

ently plugged tube that does not respond to any of these measures should be brought to the attention of the physician. An infant or small child may have to be bundled for comfort and control by the person attempting the feeding. A pacifier should be offered with every infant feeding to allow association of sucking with relief of hunger.

After feeding, the tube should be flushed with a few cc's of air (fluid column should not be visible in the latex portion of the tube); water may be used if directed by the physician. If directed, the gastrostomy tube may be clamped (using a Hoffman clamp) after the feeding and the syringe removed. The open end of the gastrostomy tube should be covered by a dry sponge. The syringe can be washed and reused. The feeding should be held and the physician notified if the child becomes distended or is vomiting.

V. Parent or significant other states what to do if tube becomes dislodged.

If the tubing becomes dislodged, the site should be covered with clean gauze taped tightly to the abdomen to decrease leakage. The patient should be brought to an emergency room as soon as possible so a physician may replace it. If the tube is out for more than a few hours, the site closes partially so that the physician might not be able to reinsert the tube. The parents should bring the dislodged tube with them to guide the physician in the selection of a new tube. Accidental dislodgement of the gastrostomy tubing is not usually painful or bloody since the wound area is usually old and healed.

VI. Parent or significant other lists items required for dressing change and feeding:
   A. Dressing change
      1. Four 1-inch-wide adhesive strips 3 inches long—2 of these split in half lengthwise
      2. Benzoin and applicator sticks
      3. Two 2 × 2-inch gauze sponges folded to 1 × 1 inch and cut in a Y shape
      4. Warm water, mild soap, towel
   B. Feeding
      1. 60-cc irrigating syringe
      2. Measuring cup
      3. Hoffman clamp
      4. Feeding preparation

Teaching Resources

Diagram of anatomy of stomach
Demonstration of wound site and care by nurse
Demonstration of feeding by nurse

BIBLIOGRAPHY

Fochtman, D., & Reffensperger, J.G. (1976). *Principles of nursing care for the pediatric surgery patient* (2nd ed.) Boston: Little, Brown & Co.

	Content/ Reinforcement Delivered	Learner Objectives Met	Not Applicable
	Date & RN	Date & RN	

INFANT GAVAGE FEEDING

Purpose

To ensure that parents can safely gavage feed their infant at home.

Content

    I. Need for infant gavage feeding
    II. Basic anatomy of the upper gastrointestinal tract
    III. Proper mouth care
    IV. Description of thrush
    V. Procedural steps for inserting the feeding tube
    VI. Procedure for feeding the infant via gavage
    VII. Removal of the gavage tube
    VIII. Reuse of gavage tube and storage of equipment

Learner Objectives

    I. The parents describe the reasons for gavage feeding their infant.

    II. The parents describe the basic anatomy of the upper gastrointestinal tract:
      A. Nasopharnyx
      B. Esophagus
      C. Stomach
      The nasopharnyx opens downward; the esophagus leads to the opening of the stomach, which is just below the xyphoid process (see Figure 3).
    III. The parents demonstrate proper mouth care, which includes cleansing the nares and mouth with cotton swabs and warm water to keep mucous membranes moist and free of irritation.
    IV. The parents define thrush, how to check for it, and who is to be notified if it is discovered.
      A. Thrush is white patches seen along the sides of the mouth or tongue; they cannot be removed by gentle rubbings with a cotton swab.
      B. During feedings, the mouth should be checked for thrush.
      C. Pediatrician should be notified if thrush is discovered.

	Content/ Reinforcement Delivered Date & RN	Learner Objectives Met Date & RN	Not Applicable

V. The parents demonstrate insertion of the feeding tube and proper mouth care three times.
  A. They name and assemble proper equipment:
    1. Disposable gavage set and appropriate size nasogastric tube
    2. 3-cc syringe
    3. Stethoscope
    4. Feeding (warmed if refrigerated)
    5. Pacifier, if appropriate
    6. Blanket
    7. Pink tape or nonallergic tape, which can be purchased outside the hospital and cut to ½-inch width
    8. Cotton swabs moistened with warm water
  B. Insert and secure the tube.
    1. Place infant on back and measure insertion length of feeding tube.
      a) *Oral*. Measure from base of nares to the distal end of the xyphoid. Mark this spot with piece of tape.
      b) *Nasal*. Measure from the tip of the nose to the midear and from midear to the xyphoid. Mark this spot with a piece of tape.
    2. Advance the tubing to the spot marked with tape. Observe for curling of the tube in pharynx.
    3. Tape tube to the side of the mouth or upper lip.
    4. If baby is active, wrap the patient in a blanket before inserting tube.
  C. Check for proper tube placement.
    1. Fill syringe with 1.5 to 2 cc of air and connect to feeding tube.
    2. Place stethoscope over infant's stomach and rapidly instill air. Listen for pop. Withdraw air instilled.
    3. Aspirate gastric contents. Note character and amount. Replace what was aspirated.
VI. The parents demonstrate the procedure for gavage feeding their infant three times.
  A. Begin the feeding properly
    1. Position baby on side or with head up.
    2. Fill the gavage syringe and tubing with feeding.
    3. Connect gavage set to feeding tube. Milk latex tubing to start flow if necessary.
  B. Regulate the rate of flow
    1. 2 cc per minute for small infant
    2. 4 cc per minute for an older infant
  C. Holding the infant comfortably
    1. Hold infant closely.
    2. Offer pacifier if appropriate.			

	Content/ Reinforcement Delivered Date & RN	Learner Objectives Met Date & RN	Not Applicable

3. Feed in quiet, relaxed atmosphere; talk to infant.
D. State hazards to watch for during feeding and proper action to follow
   1. Blood- or bile-tinged residual before feeding. Remove tube and notify physician.
   2. Infant gags or becomes restless during feed. Pinch feeding tube and allow rest period.
   3. Infant spits, vomits, or changes color. Pinch feeding tube and remove it.
VII. The parents demonstrate removal of feeding tube and proper positioning of infant after feeding three times.
  A. Pinch feeding tube in half and remove it.
  B. Position child on stomach or side.
VIII. The parents state cleaning and storage procedure for equipment.
  A. Gavage set and feeding tube may be used three to four times or until milk curds cannot be removed from tubing.
   1. Clean gavage set, feeding tube, and syringe with warm water.
   2. Flush tubing with air to remove all water.
   3. Store all equipment in clean towel.			

Evaluation If parent or significant others are unable to complete some or all of this teaching plan, document evaluation in progress notes.			

Figure 3 The Upper Gastrointestinal Tract

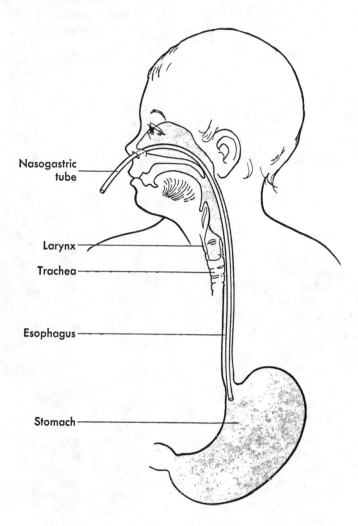

	Content/ Reinforcement Delivered	Learner Objectives Met	Not Applicable
	Date & RN	Date & RN	

OSTOMY CARE

Purpose

To educate the ostomy patients so they can maintain stoma and peristomal skin integrity.

Content

    I. Stoma (state type of stoma)
    II. Purpose of appliance
    III. How to measure for appliance size
    IV. How to assemble appliance
    V. When appliance should be changed
    VI. Steps of stoma and peristomal skin care
    VII. How to order supplies once discharged
    VIII. Contacting doctor or ostomy nurse

Learner Objectives

    I. The patient defines a stoma and its function.

    II. The patient describes the purpose of the appliance.

    III. The patient describes and demonstrates how to measure the stoma for a proper fitting appliance.
       A. The patient demonstrates use of a stoma guide to measure the stoma.
       B. The patient cuts stoma-adhesive to the exact size of the stoma. (Stoma-adhesive should "hug" a urostomy or ileostomy stoma.)
       C. The patient states that appliance with a hard disc or ring should be obtained $\frac{1}{16}$-inch or $\frac{1}{8}$-inch size larger than stoma size to prevent the ring from cutting the stoma.
    IV. The patient describes and demonstrates how to assemble the appliance. (These steps are used for urostomies and also with ostomies with excess liquid excreta.)

	Content/ Reinforcement Delivered Date & RN	Learner Objectives Met Date & RN	Not Applicable
A. Using stoma guide, the patient demonstrates how to draw a circle and cut the circle out in the center of the stoma-adhesive (circle should be the same size as the stoma).			
B. The patient removes the paper backing. The karaya ring is removed from urinary bags only, because urine breaks down karaya.			
C. The patient places stoma-adhesives (shiny side up) on a flat surface. The pouch is centered over the stoma-adhesive and is applied by gently pressing it onto the stoma-adhesive, smoothing out any wrinkles. The patient states that if wrinkles are present, there will be a tunnel through which stool or urine can flow, causing leakage (a cause of skin irritation).			
V. The patient states when the appliance should be changed*:			
A. When it leaks			
B. At least every 5 days			
C. Not more than once a day unless there is a leaking problem			
D. Daily to inspect the skin, if the skin is irritated			
VI. The patient describes and demonstrates steps of stoma and peristomal skin care.			
A. The patient empties the appliance into the toilet or a container before removing the appliance.			
B. The patient demonstrates how to remove appliance with care to prevent skin trauma.			
1. Gently push down on skin as tape is pulled away from skin.			
2. Use water to help loosen adhesive, if necessary, and states that solvents are also available.			
C. The patient wipes away waste and karaya buildup from the stoma and peristomal area with tissues or toilet paper.			
D. The patient demonstrates how to wash the stoma and peristomal area using a mild soap and warm water, and states that the use of deodorant soap may disturb the normal skin flora, resulting in a rash or irritation.			
E. The patient rinses and drys the skin well and states that the appliance will not adhere to a wet surface.			
F. The patient states that if the peristomal area appears reddened or irritated mycostatin powder should be applied.			

*Helpful hint. A shower with the bag off at the time the bag is changed will keep the skin in good condition. It is not mandatory to remove the bag each time a shower or bath is taken.

	Content/ Reinforcement Delivered Date & RN	Learner Objectives Met Date & RN	Not Applicable
1. States that a small amount of the powder is applied to the skin surface and rubbed in well.			
2. Explains that too much powder will prevent the appliance from adhering to the skin.			
3. States that if a rash extends to an area not covered by tape, mycostatin powder should be applied two times a day.			
G. The patient demonstrates how to apply a very thin layer of skin gel or similar product to the area covered by the appliance and states that the skin gel is effective for preventing irritation associated with repeated use of adhesives.			
H. The patient demonstrates application of a bag.			
1. Pulls the skin above the stoma taut with the flat of the hand (so the abdomen appears smooth).			
2. Centers the appliance over the stoma and applies it, gently pressing with the fingers.			
3. Smooths out the remaining adhesive so no wrinkles are present.			
I. The patient secures the bottom of the appliance with a plug or clamp.			
J. The patient demonstrates how the belt attaches the appliance to the body.			
1. States that the belt gives the appliance less freedom of movement.			
2. Describes how the belt will help with a leaking appliance.			
VII. The patient describes method of obtaining supplies.			
A. The patient demonstrates how to remeasure the stoma before ordering to check the size.			
1. States that it takes 6 to 8 weeks after surgery for a stoma to shrink in size.			
2. States the stoma should be remeasured periodically to check for changes.			
B. The patient states the phone number of the local supplier and the stock numbers of supplies needed to be ordered.			
C. The patient checks with the insurance company about coverage for ostomy supplies.			
1. States that most insurance companies will reimburse 80% of ostomy supplies.			
2. States that sales slips must be submitted for reimbursement.			
VIII. The patient describes the reasons for contacting the ostomy nurse or doctor:			
A. Skin irritation			

	Content/ Reinforcement Delivered Date & RN	Learner Objectives Met Date & RN	Not Applicable

1. Describes how the skin around the stoma should be inspected each time the appliance is changed.
2. States that skin irritation is slightly reddish skin or a rash around the stoma, which, if untreated, will become red, weeping, excoriated areas.
3. States if a skin irritation does not start to clear within 48 hours of proper stoma care, a physician should be contacted for advice.
B. Excessive swelling of the stoma, a change in stoma coloring, or excessive bleeding around or from the stoma. States that a small amount of bleeding when the bag is changed is not unusual. If bleeding persists, a doctor should be called.
C. Obstruction
  1. States that constipation that cannot be relieved by stool softeners (i.e., Colace and Surfak) or irrigation may be sign of obstruction.
  2. States that a physician should be notified in case of severe constipation accompanied by nausea, cramps, or vomiting.
  3. States if there is a marked change in bowel habits, either diarrhea or constipation, the physician will be notified.			

Evaluation If patient or significant others are unable to complete some or all of this teaching plan, document evaluation in progress notes.			

Part IV

The Genitourinary System

	Content/ Reinforcement Delivered Date & RN	Learner Objectives Met Date & RN	Not Applicable

HEMODIALYSIS
 	
Purpose
 	
To decrease the patient's anxiety about renal disease and the process of hemodialysis.
 	
Content
 	
  I. The function of the kidneys in health
  II. Basic renal anatomy and physiology
  III. The function of the kidneys in disease
  IV. Renal failure—acute versus chronic
  V. Etiology of renal failure—individual disease process
  VI. Symptoms of renal failure
  VII. Intervention with hemodialysis
 VIII. Hemodialysis—understanding the procedure
  IX. Concepts of diffusion, osmosis, and ultrafiltration
  X. Implementation of home management regimen			

Learner Objectives
 	
  I. The patient describes the following major functions of the kidney in health:
    A. Eliminates waste products from the digestion of food
    B. Controls fluid balance of the body to prevent fluid overload or underload
    C. Secretes hormones that help control:
      1. Blood pressure
      2. Blood cell production
  II. The patient describes the basic renal anatomy and physiology in the following simple terms:
    A. Location. The patient points to the area below the rib cage, in back, to the left and right of the spinal column.
    B. Number. Most people have two, some have one.
    C. Function
      1. Removes excess fluid from the blood
      2. Removes poisonous waste like urea, creatinine
      3. Controls the balance of chemicals in the blood, such as potassium and sodium
    D. Blood supply
      1. To the kidney from the renal artery
      2. From kidney to the blood stream by the renal vein
    E. Nephron. The part of the kidney that actually does the work.
      1. 1,000,000 nephrons in each kidney
      2. Separates waste products and fluid from the blood			

	Content/ Reinforcement Delivered Date & RN	Learner Objectives Met Date & RN	Not Applicable

F. Elimination of excess fluid and waste products.
    1. The excess fluid with waste products that compose the urine leaves the nephron by means of two tubes called the *ureters*.
    2. Fluid is carried to the *bladder*, which stores the urine until it is eliminated from the body by *urination*.
III. The patient identifies three main renal functions that can be interrupted by kidney disease:
    A. The kidney's ability to separate and eliminate waste products. *Uremia* is the medical condition that develops when waste products are retained in the blood stream.
    B. The kidney's ability to remove extra fluid from the bloodstream. Urine production decreases or stops.
    C. The secretion of hormones. High blood pressure or anemia may result.
IV. The patient states that own renal failure is
    A. Acute. The loss of kidney function was sudden and unexpected.
    B. Chronic. The loss of renal function occurred slowly and was expected.
V. The patient states the name of own renal disease and describes, in simple terms, how it affects the kidneys
 	
(see guidelines).
VI. The patient lists the following symptoms of kidney failure and relates these symptoms to the cause:
    A. Uremic symptoms (caused because waste products remain) in the blood
        1. Itching
        2. Fatigue
        3. Weakness
        4. Nausea and vomiting
        5. Nosebleeds
        6. Mental confusion
    B. Hypertension (high blood pressure caused by retained salt and water)
    C. Edema (swelling caused by retained fluid)
        1. External. Affects the tissues of the fingers, legs, eye sockets, and lower back.
        2. Internal. Affects the tissues of the lung and can cause shortness of breath.			

	Content/ Reinforcement Delivered Date & RN	Learner Objectives Met Date & RN	Not Applicable
D. Anemia. Low red-blood-cell count. The kidney cannot make the hormone needed to allow new blood cells to be formed.			
VII. The patient states dialysis may be initiated for the following reasons:			
A. An increase in uremic symptoms such as nausea, itching			
B. Toxic substances in the blood (potassium, creatinine, urea, nitrogen)			
C. Uncontrollable high blood pressure			
D. Excess fluid in the extremities or lungs			
E. Pericardial effusion (buildup of fluid in the sac that surrounds the heart)			
VIII. The patient describes the hemodialysis equipment and procedure:			
A. Equipment			
1. Artificial kidney			
a. Acts as a filter to remove waste and fluids from the blood.			
b. Holds ½ cup of blood.			
c. The inside has a membrane with tiny holes that allow water and waste products to flow out, yet keep important blood cells and protein inside.			
2. Blood tubing. A plastic tube that carries blood from the patient's access site to the artificial kidney.			
3. Dialysis machine. Controls the rate at which waste products and extra fluid can be removed from the blood.			
B. Procedure			
1. Blood circulates through the artificial kidney on one side of a membrane.			
2. A special chemical solution, *dialysate,* circulates on the opposite side of the membrane.			
3. The dialysate acts as a magnet to attract fluid and waste products out of the blood and into the dialysate.			
4. The dialysate is discarded after it flows through the artificial kidney.			
5. Approximately 1 cup of blood is in the artificial kidney and blood tubing at any one time. After it circulates in the artificial kidney, it is returned to the bloodstream.			
6. Blood constantly circulates through the artificial kidney during the hours the patient is connected to the machine.			
7. The doctor decides how many hours/treatment and treatments/week are needed.			

	Content/ Reinforcement Delivered Date & RN	Learner Objectives Met Date & RN	Not Applicable

8. Unless the doctor orders it, there is no blood transfusion during dialysis.
IX. The patient gives a simple explanation of the concepts of diffusion, osmosis, and ultrafiltration:
  A. Diffusion. The dialysate acts like a magnet to attract toxic wastes out of the blood, where their level is high, and into the dialysate, where their level is low.
  B. Osmosis. The blood has more water in it than does the dialysate, so water will leave the bloodstream and go into the dialysate in an effort to dilute it.
  C. Ultrafiltration. When too much weight is gained from fluid intake, pressure can be applied to one side of the membrane in the artificial kidney to push extra water out of the blood and into the dialysate.
X. The patient demonstrates ability to safely implement home management regimen between treatments.
  1. The patient states the procedure to follow in order to contact: the physician, dialysis unit, and emergency room.
  2. The patient states the prescribed diet:
    _____protein
    _____potassium
    _____calcium
    _____cc fluid/24 hours
  3. The patient states dialysis schedule. _____
  4. The patient meets the objectives of the medication teaching plan.
  5. The patient demonstrates the correct use of a scale.
  6. The patient determines the correct pre- and postdialysis weights. _____
  7. The patient demonstrates procedure for preparation of access sites predialysis (see teaching guides for arteriovenous shunts and arteriovenous fistulas and grafts).		

Evaluation If patient or significant others are unable to complete part or all of this teaching plan, document evaluation in progress notes.		

GUIDELINES: HEMODIALYSIS

A patient beginning a hemodialysis program should be given a thorough explanation of the hemodialysis procedure. The nurse must assess the patient's capability for learning. Uremia causes lassitude and disorientation. Formal teaching is started when physiological equilibrium is restored.

If the teaching guide is initiated by a nurse on an inpatient unit, a hemodialysis nurse should be involved. A tour of the hemodialysis unit should be arranged. This teaching guide should be used in conjunction with the teaching guides for A-V fistula and graft and A-V shunts and should be completed before starting teaching for self-care dialysis if appropriate.

II. Renal anatomy and physiology in health. The kidneys are located on either side of the vertebral column in the posterior portion of the abdominal cavity. Most people have two kidneys, though some may have only one or as many as three. The single unit of the kidney is the nephron. There are approximately 1 million nephrons in each kidney. The nephron surrounds a capillary bed called the *glomerulus*. The glomerulus acts as the filtering unit of the kidney. As blood passes through the glomerulus, metabolic end products and body fluids are selectively filtered out and excreted from the body as urine.

The kidneys are also responsible for releasing hormones that help control blood pressure and red blood cell production.

IV. Acute versus chronic renal failure. Acute renal failure is a rapid deterioration of kidney function that occurs in a matter of hours or days. This may be due to severe shock, hemorrhage, chemical or drug poisoning, glomerulonephritis, injury or obstruction of the blood vessels leading to the kidneys. In most cases of acute renal failure, normal kidney function is restored within several weeks. Dialysis is usually required for only a few weeks, but in some instances renal impairment is permanent. Chronic renal failure develops over a long period. Initial symptoms include hypertension, weakness, and anemia. These symptoms usually occur after 50% of renal function is lost. Dialysis or renal transplantation is usually required when 90% of renal function is lost. Chronic renal failure may be caused by an inherited disease such as polycystic kidney disease or by an acquired disease such as glomerulonephritis or diabetes.

To the nurse: Most patients with chronic renal failure have lived with their disease for a long time. They may not, however, really understand it. The level of patient knowledge must be assessed before teaching can begin. Also the nurse must be sensitive to the patients whose disease is hereditary because these patients are concerned about their families as well as themselves.

V. Etiology of renal disease. The following are examples of diseases that may cause renal failure. Use these brief explanations to help the patient understand the relationship between the individual disease process and renal failure.

A. Chronic glomerulonephritis. Glomerulonephritis is the most common cause of chronic renal failure. It is a chronic inflammation of the renal glomeruli, the small filtering units of the kidney. This impairs the kidney's ability to filter large molecules such as protein. The inflammation is often the result of the body's response to a bacterial infection or exposure to some chemicals, but sometimes the etiology is unknown. The body's attempt to destroy a streptococcal respiratory tract infection commonly precedes glomerulonephritis.

B. Nephrotic syndrome (hydronephrosis, nephrosis). Nephrotic syndrome is the result of an increased loss of plasma proteins (albumin) through the renal glomeruli. It is caused by diseases that affect the glomeruli, for example, glomerulonephritis, or diseases that affect the systemic blood vessels, for example, diabetic neuropathy. Occasionally nephrotic syndrome is associated with allergic reactions.

The major symptom is massive body swelling. The patient also usually has protein in the urine, a low albumin level in the blood, and an increased lipid level in the blood. Other symptoms are those associated with acute renal failure.

Treatment is nonspecific and is aimed at the relief of symptoms and the prevention of complications. If the underlying cause of nephrotic syndrome is reversible, the chance of cure or remission is good. If the nature of the underlying disease is irreversible, terminal renal failure results.

C. Pyelonephritis. Pyelonephritis is an acute or chronic bacterial infection of the kidney. With repeated infections, areas of scar tissue develop and inflammation occurs. This leads to the destruction of kidney tissue. The kidney cannot perform its normal function, and uremia often occurs. Symptoms of pyelonephritis include back pain, fever, painful burning during urination, frequency of urination, and pus in the urine. Treatment is aimed at clearing up the infection and relieving the patient's pain.

D. Diabetic nephropathy. Patients with longstanding and poorly controlled diabetes can eventually have renal deterioration. This is caused by systemic vascular changes that lead to the deterioration of the glomeruli and the development of uremia.

E. Lupus erythematosis. Lupus erythematosis, a collagen disease, destroys the area around the glomerulus called the *basement membrane,* which is comprised of collagen. This leads to glomerular swelling, scarring, and renal failure. Large doses of steroid medication are administered to the patient in order to slow down the progression of the disease, but chronic renal failure often develops.

VI. Symptoms of renal failure. Should the kidneys fail to function normally, uremia, hypertension, edema, and anemia may result. Uremia is a condition caused by the buildup of metabolic end products in the bloodstream. Symptoms of uremia include weakness, fatigability, vomiting, nausea, generalized itching, and sleep disturbances. Symptoms of severe uremia are nosebleed, gastrointestinal bleeding, impaired memory, confusion, and emotional instability. Hypertension and edema may develop from circulatory overload due to the kidney's inability to regulate body fluids. Anemia may result from the kidney's inability to secrete the hormone necessary to stimulate red blood cell production. This hormone is called *erythropoietin.*

VII. Hemodialysis procedure. During hemodialysis an artificial kidney is utilized to mimic the two major functions of the normal kidney: clearance of toxins and elimination of excess body water. It is composed of a semipermeable membrane encased in a hard plastic shell. Blood is carried from the patient by special blood tubing attached to the patient's access site. The dialysis machine controls the speed at which blood is circulated through the artificial kidney. It also controls the flow of a special chemical solution called *dialysate*. In the artificial kidney, blood flows on one side of the semipermeable membrane while the dialysate flows simultaneously along the other side.

During dialysis, the following three processes occur:

1. Diffusion. Diffusion is the movement of particles from a solution of high concentration to a solution of low concentration.
2. Osmosis. Osmosis is the passage of fluid through a semipermeable membrane (separating fluids of different concentrations) from the solution of lower concentration to the solution of higher concentration.
3. Ultrafiltration. Ultrafiltration is an applied force to one side of a semipermeable membrane to enhance the process of osmosis.

During dialysis, metabolic end products are filtered from the blood stream by osmosis. Excess fluid is withdrawn by the application of ultrafiltration.

	Content/ Reinforcement Delivered Date & RN	Learner Objectives Met Date & RN	Not Applicable

ARTERIOVENOUS FISTULAS AND GRAFTS

Purpose

To enable patients to participate in their health care by educating them about their access site.

To teach patients to react quickly and accurately in an emergency situation involving their access site.

Content

   I. General anatomy and physiology of an arteriovenous fistula or a graft

  II. Exercises to enhance fistula development

 III. Physical restrictions

 IV. Complications of fistulas and grafts

  V. Signs and symptoms, preventive and restorative action related to complications

 VI. Explanation and demonstration of skin care

Learner Objectives

   I. Patient describes basic anatomy and physiology of access site:

     A. Arteriovenous fistula

       1. This is created by sewing an artery to a nearby vein and making one blood vessel.

       2. Blood from the heart (arterial) will mix with blood returning to the heart (venous).

       3. Mixing arterial and venous blood together will cause the vessel to enlarge. This process, called *arterialization,* takes place within 4 to 6 weeks.

       4. After arterialization, needles can be temporarily placed into the fistula to allow access to the blood stream for dialysis.

       5. Patient states location of fistula.

     B. Graft. Patient states type and shows location of graft:

       1. Gortex

          a) Synthetic tube of material is sewn between an artery and vein to make an artificial arterialized vein.

          b) Patient states reason for graft, "My own blood vessels are inadequate because of size or disease."

          c) A Gortex graft can be used after 10 days.

       2. Umbilical vein graft

          a) A section of human umbilical vein is sewn between an artery and vein to create an artificial arterialized vein.

	Content/ Reinforcement Delivered Date & RN	Learner Objectives Met Date & RN	Not Applicable
b) Patient states reason for using an umbilical vein graft as "because my own vessels are inadequate because of size or disease or because I am allergic to the material in a Gortex graft."			
c) An umbilical vein graft can be used after 10 days.			
II. Patient demonstrates proper exercises to enhance development of an arteriovenous fistula.			
A. Patient demonstrates proper placement of tourniquet on a nonaccess site extremity.			
B. Patient demonstrates the following exercises:			
1. Place tourniquet above fistula and clench and relax hand for 1 minute, then remove tourniquet. Do four times daily. If pain in hand from tourniquet is not tolerable, immediately release tourniquet.			
2. Place tourniquet above fistula and alternately squeeze and release a hard rubber ball for 1 minute, then remove tourniquet. Do four times daily.			
3. If able, depending on location of fistula, immerse extremity with fistula into warm water and perform exercises with or without tourniquet in place.			
III. Patient lists the following restrictions of an arteriovenous fistula or graft.			
A. Avoid constrictive clothing or jewelry on extremity with access site.			
B. Avoid pressure on access site during sleep.			
C. If access site is located in arm, avoid bending that extremity for prolonged periods.			
D. Avoid compression of access site by not carrying heavy objects such as school books, purses.			
E. No blood drawing from access site except by dialysis personnel.			
F. No blood pressure measurements on access site extremity.			
IV. Patient lists the common complications of arteriovenous fistulas and grafts:			
A. Infection			
B. Hematoma			
C. Clotting			
D. Bleeding			
V. Patient describes each complication with regard to signs, symptoms, and preventative, therapeutic, or restorative action:			
A. Infection			
1. Symptoms			
a) Redness			
b) Warmth			
c) Swelling			

	Content/ Reinforcement Delivered Date & RN	Learner Objectives Met Date & RN	Not Applicable

      d) Tenderness

      e) Drainage

  2. Intervention

      a) Should any of these symptoms be noticed, the physician or dialysis nurse should be contacted immediately.

      b) The access site must be observed daily for any signs of infection.

      c) In presence of infection, antibiotics will be used.

B. Hematoma formation

  1. Symptoms

      a) Swelling

      b) Pain at needle sites

      c) Bruising (delayed sign)

  2. Interventions

      a) When hematoma is observed, immediately place firm pressure on site to stop further bleeding.

      b) When bleeding stops, apply ice to site for 10 minutes to constrict blood vessels.

      c) On day after dialysis, soak access in warm water three to four times to help reabsorb old blood.

      d) The physician or dialysis nurse must be called for any further bleeding. Telephone number to call is _____.

C. Clotting of access site

  1. Procedure for checking bruit.

      a) Check for a bruit twice a day in the morning and evening.

      b) If a change in the bruit is noticed

         (1) Call physician immediately.

         (2) Go to emergency room.

D. Excessive bleeding from access site

  1. Procedure for holding direct pressure to bleeding site to stop bleeding.

      a) If bleeding lasts more than 30 minutes, medical attention will be sought.

      b) A package of gauze will be with patient should bleeding restart.

VI. Patient demonstrates the following skin care technique:

A. Predialysis

  1. Wash hands.

  2. Cleanse area with alcohol swabs.

  3. Cleanse again with betadine swabs.

  4. Cover with sterile gauze.

B. Postdialysis

  1. Hold direct pressure over bleeding site for 10 to 15 minutes, until bleeding stops.

	Content/ Reinforcement Delivered Date & RN	Learner Objectives Met Date & RN	Not Applicable
2. Cover needle sites with bandaid. Remove bandaid next day. C. At home. Routine skin care with soap and water. **Evaluation** If patient or significant others are unable to complete part or all of this teaching plan, document evaluation in progress notes.			

	Content/ Reinforcement Delivered Date & RN	Learner Objectives Met Date & RN	Not Applicable

ARTERIOVENOUS SHUNTS

Purpose

To teach the patient preventative, therapeutic, and restorative interventions necessary to care successfully for the arteriovenous shunt at home.

Content

    I. Anatomy of shunt placement
   II. Physical restrictions
  III. Shunt infection: signs, symptoms, and management
  IV. Shunt clotting: signs, symptoms, and management
   V. Basic principles of anticoagulation therapy
  VI. Principles of shunt care
 VII. Situations requiring emergency intervention
VIII. Interventions for emergency situations

Learner Objectives

    I. The patient describes the anatomy of a shunt in simple terms.

    A. The patient points to the location of the shunt.
    B. The patient describes the shunt as
       1. An external access site to the bloodstream
       2. One plastic cannula sewn into an artery
       3. A second plastic cannula sewn into a vein
       4. Two external ends joined with a teflon connector
       5. Blood flowing from the artery through the shunt and returning back to the blood stream through the vein
   II. The patient states restrictions in the following terms:
    A. A shunt must never be opened except during dialysis by a dialysis nurse or technician.
    B. The extremity with the shunt should be elevated during rest periods until swelling is gone.
    C. Constrictive clothing or jewelry should be avoided over the shunt.
    D. Lifting or carrying heavy objects should be avoided if the shunt is in an arm.
    E. Bulldog clamps must be carried on person at all times.

	Content/ Reinforcement Delivered Date & RN	Learner Objectives Met Date & RN	Not Applicable

III. The patient states the signs and symptoms of an infected shunt and states the appropriate preventative or restorative action to take:
 	
A. Signs and symptoms
  1. Warm, red, and tender skin around the exit site
  2. Drainage or pus from exit sites
  3. Appearance of red streaks in the extremity above the shunt
  4. Pain
  5. Fever
  6. Chills
 	
B. Preventative measures
  1. Care for skin (refer to learner objective VI).
  2. Keep shunt securely bandaged during off-dialysis times.
  3. Avoid prolonged exposure to moisture. If the dressing becomes wet, change it.
 	
C. Restorative measures
  1. Report any of the preceding symptoms to the physician or dialysis nurse as soon as noted.
  2. Take antibiotics as ordered by the physician.
  3. Use meticulous skin care to avoid spreading bacteria from one exit site to the other.
 	
IV. The patient states the signs and symptoms of a clotting shunt and states the appropriate preventative or restorative action to take:
 	
A. Signs and symptoms
  1. A change in the color of blood visible in the shunt tubing from red to blue-black
  2. The presence of white flecks that may indicate clot formation
  3. A change in bruit (sound of blood as it flows through shunt and into vein)
  4. A change in the temperature of the blood in the shunt from warm to cool
 	
B. Preventative measures
  1. Check the shunt every morning and afternoon for the presence of any symptoms of clotting.
  2. Avoid tight clothes or jewelry over the shunt.
  3. Avoid kinking the shunt tubing during bandaging.
  4. Avoid prolonged exposure to cold.
  5. Never place a tourniquet above the shunt.
  6. No blood pressure measurement should be taken in the shunt extremity.
  7. No venipuncture should be done in the shunt extremity.		

	Content/ Reinforcement Delivered Date & RN	Learner Objectives Met Date & RN	Not Applicable

C. Should shunt clotting be suspected, the patient will
  1. Immediately notify the physician.
  2. Go immediately to the dialysis unit during working hours.
  3. Go immediately to an emergency room if the dialysis unit is closed and state, "I suspect that my shunt may be clotting."

V. The patient states reasons why an anticoagulant is needed and describes the proper regimen for taking it.
  A. Intervention with anticoagulant is necessary when
    1. There is repeated shunt clotting.
    2. There is a shunt with poor arterial flow predisposed to clotting.
  B. The patient meets objectives of the medication teaching plan for the anticoagulant drug.
  C. The patient states that the following will be reported *immediately*:
    1. Any bleeding—from stomach, nose, stool, or urine
    2. Bruising (can indicate bleeding has occurred)
    3. Abdominal or joint pain
    4. Severe headaches

VI. Following a demonstration, the patient demonstrates the correct procedure for cleaning and bandaging an arteriovenous shunt:
  A. Cleaning
    1. Wash hands.
    2. Remove old dressing.
    3. For each exit site:
      a) Wash with alcohol swabs.
      b) Follow by wash with iodine swabs.
      c) Pat dry with sterile gauze.
      d) A separate swab must be used for each exit site to avoid transmitting germs from one exit site to the other.
    4. Remove crusting or exudate from exit sites.
      a. Moisten a sterile gauze with hydrogen peroxide.
      b. Gently clean around the exit site.
      c. Use a separate sterile gauze pad for each exit site.
  B. Bandaging procedure
    1. Place a sterile 4×4 gauze under the loop of the shunt.
    2. Place a sterile 4×4 gauze over the exit sites.
    3. Open a sterile 4×4 gauze square and lay it flat across the shunt; secure both ends with tape.
    4. Cover with a "kling" gauze, wrapped securely, but not tightly, in figure-8 fashion.

	Content/ Reinforcement Delivered Date & RN	Learner Objectives Met Date & RN	Not Applicable

5. Leave a small portion of the loop visible to allow observation for shunt clotting.
VII. The patient states potential situations that would require emergency intervention:
  A. Shunt separation at the connection site
  B. Dislodgement of the teflon tubing from the exit site
 	
VIII. The patient states the cause, risk, and intervention necessary if a shunt comes apart at the connector, i.e., is dislodged from exit site:
  A. Separation of shunt at connector
    1. Cause. Poor fit between shunt tubing and connector—accidental pulling on one side of shunt.
    2. Risk. Hemorrhage or infection
    3. Intervention
      a) Immediately clamp both ends of the shunt (patient demonstrates correct use of bulldog clamps).
      b) Proceed immediately to an emergency room.
  B. Dislodgement of the shunt tubing from the exit site.
    1. Cause
      a) Accidental pulling of shunt tubing out of skin
      b) Poor tissue integrity from repeated infection
      c) Skin breakdown around exit site
    2. Risk. Hemorrhage (severe) or infection
    3. Intervention
      a) Dislodgement of the arterial end
        (1) Apply direct pressure to the exit site to stop bleeding.
        (2) Clamp the venous end of the shunt to stop bleeding.
        (3) If direct pressure does not stop the bleeding, apply a tourniquet above the shunt.
        (4) Go directly to an emergency room.
      b) Dislodgement of the venous end
        (1) Clamp the arterial end of shunt.
        (2) Apply direct pressure to the venous exit site.
        (3) Proceed immediately to an emergency room.
 	
Evaluation
 	
If patient or significant others are unable to complete some or all of this teaching plan, document evaluation in progress notes.		

GUIDELINES: ARTERIOVENOUS SHUNTS

I. An arteriovenous shunt provides direct access to a person's bloodstream to allow the hemodialysis procedure to occur.

    A surgeon implants one tip of the shunt into an artery and the other end into a vein. The external portions of the two shunt ends are joined with a tight-fitting teflon connector. Subsequently blood flows from the artery through the shunt into the vein and back to the bloodstream.

    To begin hemodialysis, the dialysis nurse opens the shunt and attaches the arterial and venous ends to the arterial and venous blood lines on the dialysis machine. When the dialysis procedure is completed, the shunt is closed and rebandaged.

    Shunts are most commonly placed in a nondominant extremity; often the radial artery and brachial vein are used. Vascular difficulties may necessitate alternate site selection.

III. Infection is a very serious hazard to the life of both the shunt and the patient. Meticulous care of the shunt by both patients and staff is essential. The patient must be instructed to observe the shunt carefully for any signs or symptoms of infection and report any findings to the dialysis nurse or to the physician.

    Because a shunt provides direct access to the heart, bacterial endocarditis can develop as a complication of shunt infection. For this reason, all shunt infections must be adequately treated with a full course of antibiotics, usually lasting 6 weeks.

    Osteomyelitis is another serious complication that can develop from an infected shunt. The seeding of infection to bone is extremely dangerous, and patients with this problem are hospitalized for intravenous antibiotics.

    Repeated infections also destroy the integrity of the skin around the exit site of the shunt, making the accidental dislodgment or erosion of the shunt through the skin a distinct possibility.

    The patient must understand the very real danger of shunt infections. Infections resistant to treatment necessitate shunt removal. The shunt is the patient's lifeline to the dialysis machine; there are limited body areas suitable for shunt placement.

IV. As soon as a shunt is inserted, a patient should be taught to observe it for clotting. If the patient is too anxious or uremic to comprehend the instruction, a family member or significant other should be taught. Declotting a shunt must never be attempted except by a dialysis nurse or physician. Quick action when clotting is suspected will enhance the chances for successful declotting.

V. In some cases of repeated shunt clotting episodes, anticoagulants may be used. Aspirin is the drug of choice, but sometimes Coumadin is used. Patients must be fully instructed about these drugs and the risks of anticoagulation treatment.

VI. The nurse should explain and demonstrate the procedure for cleaning and bandaging a shunt. The patient should be gradually given responsibility for the difficult steps in the procedure, so that eventually the patient is performing the entire procedure. Periodic checks of the patient's routine will ascertain that the procedure is being done correctly.

    Again, if the nurse determines that the patient will require assistance or supervision to perform the procedure correctly, a family member or significant other should be included in the teaching plan.

	Content/ Reinforcement Delivered Date & RN	Learner Objectives Met Date & RN	Not Applicable

RENAL TRANSPLANT

Purpose

To help the patient make an informed decision regarding renal transplantation.
To reduce the apprehension and increase the cooperation of the pretransplant patient.

Content

    I. Factors to be considered for a renal transplant
   II. Anatomy and physiology of the kidney
  III. Pathophysiology of patient's kidney disease
  IV. Transplant criteria
   V. Principles related to blood and tissue typing
  VI. Preoperative tests and procedures
 VII. Factors to consider for a living relative donor
VIII. Factors to consider for a cadaver donor
  IX. Success rate of transplantation
   X. Preoperative procedures
  XI. Operative procedures
 XII. Postoperative events
XIII. Signs and symptoms of rejection
XIV. Medication
 XV. Dialysis after transplantation
XVI. Home care
XVII. How to contact the physician

Learner Objectives

  I. The patient describes the factors that are considered when deciding whether to have a renal transplant.
    A. A kidney coming from a living relative is best because there is less likelihood of rejection.
    B. The patient has a greater chance to reject a kidney from a cadaver.
    C. The patient may decide to stay on dialysis if a kidney transplant is not desired.
    D. The primary decision to have kidney transplant is made by the patient.
    E. The physician and the nurse advise and help clarify questions that the patient may have regarding renal transplants.

	Content/ Reinforcement Delivered	Learner Objectives Met	Not Applicable
	Date & RN	Date & RN	

II. The patient describes the anatomy and physiology of the kidney.
   A. The two kidneys in the body are located in the lower back on each side of the spinal column just above the waistline.
   B. The kidney helps to maintain the body's chemical balance in four ways:
      1. Filters excess fluid from the body
      2. Filters waste products from the body
      3. Retains fluids and chemicals needed by the body
      4. Releases into the bloodstream hormones that help control blood pressure and blood production

III. The patient discusses the pathology associated with the kidney problem

(refer to hemodialysis teaching plan).

IV. The patient describes the pretransplantation criteria. To be a candidate for a transplant, the patient must be in good health. Generally patients should be 65 years old or younger.

V. The patient describes principles related to blood and tissue typing.
   A. Blood is typed according to the following criteria:
      1. A patient with type-O blood is a universal donor (may give blood to anyone).
      2. A patient with type-O blood can receive only O blood.
      3. A patient with type-AB blood can give only to a patient who has type-AB blood.
      4. A patient with type-AB blood is the universal recipient (may receive blood from anyone).
      5. A patient with type-A blood can give blood to a patient with type-A and type-AB blood.
      6. A patient with type-B blood can give only to a patient with type-B and type-AB blood.
   B. Tissue is typed using the following criteria:
      1. Tissue typing determines the degree of tissue compatibility between donor and recipient.
      2. The degree of rejection is affected by exposure to viral or bacterial infection, blood transfusions, pregnancy, etc.

	Content/ Reinforcement Delivered Date & RN	Learner Objectives Met Date & RN	Not Applicable

VI. The patient describes preoperative tests, procedures, and conferences.
  A. Mixed lymphocyte count (MLC) is drawn. This is a more defined blood test that will determine how close a match there is in a kidney that is received from a relative.
  B. Other routine tests include
    1. Upper GI series. The patient swallows barium to outline any abnormalities of the GI system.
    2. Chest x-ray.
    3. EKG.
    4. Routine blood and urine studies.
    5. Barium enema (scheduled if there is a history of rectal bleeding).
    6. Stool (to test for blood).
  C. A patient with heart disease may have a heart monitor stress test and a test to determine the pumping action of the heart.
  D. Blood transfusions may be necessary for the patient to receive from the relative who will be donating the kidney.
  E. Bladder function studies are sometimes ordered for the patient receiving the kidney.
  F. Arrangements are made so the patient can see the social worker who will be involved in care.
  G. A family conference is arranged when the patient decides on a renal transplant.
VII. The patient describes factors to consider for living relatives who wish to donate a kidney.
  A. The living relative must have certain tests to determine health.
    1. Blood work and a urine test are done and reviewed by the physician.
    2. An x-ray of the kidney and an arteriogram (dye injected into the kidney) are ordered.
    3. The physician reviews the information and orders other tests if necessary.
    4. The doctor schedules admission to the hospital when the renal transplant is ready to take place.
VIII. The patient describes the requirements for a cadaveric transplant.
  A. If a patient has been evaluated and found to be a candidate to receive a kidney transplant but a living relative's kidney is not possible, the patient is placed on a waiting list for a cadaveric transplant.
    1. The waiting time for a kidney may be 3 months to 4 years, depending on the antibody level.			

	Content/ Reinforcement Delivered	Learner Objectives Met	Not Applicable
	Date & RN	Date & RN	
2. Surgery occurs within 24 to 48 hours after the kidney becomes available. The new kidney is kept alive by a perfusion machine or by ice packing.			
IX. The patient describes the success rate of kidney transplantation.			
A. A kidney from a brother or sister has a success rate of 90 to 95% if there is a full tissue match.			
B. Parents or children are usually "half match" and the success range is 80 to 85%. With pretransplant blood transfusions from the donor, the success rate can be improved.			
X. The patient describes the preoperative procedure for renal transplantation.			
A. See preoperative teaching plan.			
B. If the transplant is a scheduled admission, the patient will have dialysis 2 consecutive days before surgery.			
XI. The patient explains the operative procedure.			
A. The skin incision is made in either the right or left side of the lower abdomen.			
B. The transplanted kidney is placed into the pelvis for convenience.			
C. The kidney's main artery and vein are surgically connected to the large vein and artery of the pelvis.			
D. The tube that carries urine from the kidney to the bladder is also transplanted.			
E. This tube is surgically connected to the patient's bladder.			
XII. The patient describes the postoperative events after transplant.			
A. The patient will be in the recovery room for the first 24 hours, where a nurse will monitor vital signs closely.			
B. When stable, the patient will be transferred to the floor, where the primary nurse will be introduced to the patient.			
C. Important things the nurse will monitor include			
1. Urine output			
2. Blood pressure			
3. Respiratory care			
4. Electrolyte values. BUN, Creatinine, etc.			
XIII. The patient describes the signs and symptoms of rejection:			
A. General malaise and loss of appetite			
B. Chills and increase in temperature			
C. Swelling at the surgical site			
D. Decrease in urine output			
E. Increase in blood pressure			
F. Increase in weight			
G. Increase in blood urea nitrogen and creatinine			

	Content/ Reinforcement Delivered	Learner Objectives Met	Not Applicable
	Date & RN	Date & RN	

XIV. The patient describes common medications after renal transplant (refer to medication teaching plan for the following):
  A. Imuran
  B. Prednisone
  C. Atgam
  D. Cyclosporin A
XV. The patient describes dialysis after transplant.
  A. At times temporary dialysis may be needed after the transplant. It is important to understand that this is not a bad sign.
XVI. The patient describes care of self at home after transplant.
  A. A log book is given to the patient on discharge from the hospital. In this book the patient will record daily
    1. Temperature
    2. Blood pressure
    3. Weight
    4. 24-hour intake and output
  B. The patient will also record the following in the log book:
    1. Signs and symptoms of rejection
    2. Medications taken, time administered, and side effects observed
    3. The appropriate health professionals to contact if there is a problem
XVII. The patient states how to contact the following professionals involved in care:
  A. Primary nurse
  B. Surgeon
  C. Renal medical fellow
  D. Social worker
  E. Dialysis unit
  F. Clinic nurse			

Evaluation If patient or significant others are unable to complete some or all of this teaching plan, document evaluation in progress notes.			

Part V

The Musculoskeletal System

	Content/ Reinforcement Delivered Date & RN	Learner Objectives Met Date & RN	Not Applicable

BANKHART PROCEDURE

Purpose

To familiarize the patient with aspects of surgery in order to diminish preoperative anxiety and enlist the patient's cooperation during the postoperative period.

Content

I. Brief discussion of the surgical procedure and its purpose
II. Review of the general preoperative teaching plan
III. Description of skin preparation
IV. Routine after surgery
V. Reasons to contact the physician
VI. How to contact the physician
VII. Follow-up

Learner Objectives

I. The patient describes the Bankhart procedure and its purpose.
   A. The shoulder joint is surrounded by a capsule including ligaments (cords that hold the joint together) that contribute to the stability of the joint.
   B. When ligaments weaken or detach, a dislocation often occurs.
   C. The Bankhart procedure tightens and secures the shoulder muscles to prevent dislocation.
II. The patient meets the objectives of the general preoperative teaching plan.
III. The patient describes the skin preparation before surgery.
   A. Antiseptic soap scrubs are done three to four times during the 24 hours before surgery.
   B. A formal prep and shave are done in the operating room.
IV. The patient describes the routine after surgery:
   A. Positioning
      1. The head of the bed is to be up at all times.
      2. A pillow should support the area under the back and the affected forearm.
      3. The affected arm is kept close to the body.
      4. The patient is on bedrest for the first 24 hours, then progresses slowly to activity as tolerated.
   B. Dressing
      1. A bulky dressing is on the shoulder.
      2. The arm is kept close to body by a sling and ace bandages wrapped around entire chest.

	Content/ Reinforcement Delivered Date & RN	Learner Objectives Met Date & RN	Not Applicable

C. Neurovascular checks
  1. Checks are done every hour for the first 12 hours after surgery and then every 4 hours.
  2. The nurse checks the color of the fingers of the affected arm for blanching of fingertips and notes any signs of edema.
  3. The nurse checks sensation by instructing the patient to close eyes while the nurse touches the fingers to determine if sensation is present.
  4. The nurse feels hands to check for coolness or heat.
  5. The patient is asked to move all fingers and to test the hand grasp to check for decreased motion.
  6. Any numbness or tingling should be reported to the nurse.
V. The patient describes reasons to contact the physician:
A. Dislocation of the shoulder
B. Changes in color, sensation, movement
  1. Numbness, tingling
  2. Excessive swelling of the hand on the affected side (a small amount is expected)
  3. Pale or dusky fingertips
  4. Decreased movement of affected arm or hand
C. Changes in incision site
  1. Redness
  2. Tenderness
  3. Drainage
  4. Swelling
  5. Incision line separation
D. Unexplainable fever
VI. The patient describes how to contact the physician:
A. Physician's phone #: _____
B. Emergency room #: _____
C. Orthopedic clinic #: _____
VII. The patient states date and time of follow-up appointment:
  Date: _____
  Time: _____			

Evaluation If patient or significant others are unable to complete some or all of this teaching plan, document evaluation in progress notes.			

	Content/ Reinforcement Delivered Date & RN	Learner Objectives Met Date & RN	Not Applicable

CAST CARE

Purpose

To provide the patient and family with the information necessary to care for the cast and the casted extremity.

Content

   I. Purpose of the cast
  II. Cast care and care of extremity when cast is wet
 III. Cast care and care of extremity when cast is dry
 IV. Signs and symptoms that should be reported to the physician
  V. Follow-up

Learner Objectives

   I. The patient states that the cast is used to immobilize the affected part in order to
     A. Maintain the position of fracture fragments
     B. Restrict usage of and support diseased or weakened bone, joints, or muscles
     C. Prevent or correct deformities
  II. The patient describes cast care and the care of the affected extremity when the cast is wet.
     A. Expose the cast to air, without bedding, to promote drying.
     B. Handle the cast only with the palms of the hands and support with pillows to prevent indentations.
     C. Check the toes or fingers every 2 hours for movement and warmth.
     D. Rub the skin under the edges of the cast with alcohol every 2 hours.
     E. Do not bear weight on the affected extremity while the cast is wet.
 III. The patient describes care of the cast and care of the affected extremity when the cast is dry.
     A. Continue to check the toes or fingers of the affected extremities to ensure that they can be moved, felt, and are warm to touch.
     B. Continue with alcohol care as in IID and monitor the skin around the edges of the cast for redness or breakdown.
     C. Apply moleskin cut in "petals" around the rough edges of the cast to provide a smooth surface.
     D. Protect the perineal area and the back of body casts with plastic wrap when washing or moving the bowels.

	Content/ Reinforcement Delivered	Learner Objectives Met	Not Applicable
	Date & RN	Date & RN	

E. Protect the cast from getting wet by wrapping the extremity in a plastic bag when bathing, in the rain, or at the beach.

F. Clean the cast with a damp rag if excessively dirty.

G. Elevate the extremity above the level of the heart if any swelling is present.

H. Do not put any foreign article in between the cast and the skin.

IV. The patient states the signs and symptoms that should be reported to the nurse or physician immediately:

A. Circulatory impairment
1. Unrelieved or increased pain
2. Increased swelling that is not relieved with elevation
3. Changes in color of the toes or fingers of the affected extremity
4. Tingling or numbness of the extremity
5. Inability to move the toes or fingers of the affected extremity
6. Temperature change of the skin of the affected extremity

B. Potential pressure sore
1. Itching or burning under the cast
2. Unpleasant odors from under the cast
3. Drainage from under or through the cast
4. Warm area on a dry cast
5. Increased body temperature

C. Damage to the cast
1. Cracks in the cast
2. Softening of the cast

V. Patient states follow-up:
A. Appointment
Date: _____
Time: _____
B. Physician #: _____
Emergency room #: _____

Evaluation

If patient or significant others are unable to complete some or all of this teaching plan, document evaluation in progress notes.

	Content/ Reinforcement Delivered	Learner Objectives Met	Not Applicable
	Date & RN	Date & RN	

THE IMMOBILIZED PATIENT

Purpose

To prevent complications of immobility.
To ensure optimal independence.

Content

    I. Reasons for immobility
   II. Complications of immobility
  III. Strengthening exercises
  IV. Coughing and deep breathing exercises
   V. Adequate fluid intake
  VI. Positioning
 VII. Symptoms to report to the nurse
VIII. Use of elastic stockings

Learner Objectives

    I. The patient states reasons for immobility:
       A. To promote healing of a body part
       B. To decrease workload of a body part
       C. Specific reason for immobilization
   II. The patient lists at least four complications of being immobilized:
       A. Decreased circulation
       B. Lung congestion
       C. Decreased muscle tone and strength
       D. Constipation
  III. The patient states that exercises are performed to promote circulation and maintain strength and properly performs some or all of the following exercises:
       A. Abdominal strengthening
           1. Exercise No. 1
              a) The knees may be elevated.
              b) With the head of the bed flat, push the lower back into the bed as far as possible.
              c) Hold this position for a count of 5.
           2. Exercise No. 2
              a) Lying with knees bent, raise head and shoulders from the bed.
              b) Hold for a count of 5.
       B. Shoulder and arm strengthening
           1. Exercise No. 1
               a) With the bed flat, pull the body up, utilizing the trapeze.
              b) Hold this position for a count of 5.

	Content/ Reinforcement Delivered	Learner Objectives Met	Not Applicable
	Date & RN	Date & RN	

    2. Exercise No. 2
Sand bags may be held to maintain muscle tone and strength.
      a) Go through full shoulder and arm range of motion 10 times each hour.
      b) Flex and extend the arms.
      c) Push the arms away from the body and push chin toward them.
      d) Rotate the arms in a circle.

  C. Leg strengthening
    1. Plantar flexion
      a) Push the toes away from the body as far as possible.
      b) Keep the legs on the bed.
      c) Push the soles of the feet against a foot board.
    2. Dorsi flexion
      a) Keep the legs on the bed.
      b) Bring the toes as close to the legs as possible by pointing the toes toward the ceiling and then toward the head.
    3. Gluteal sets
      a) Squeeze the buttocks together as tightly as possible.
    4. Quadriceps sets
      a) Legs are straight and resting on the bed.
      b) Push the knee into the mattress as far as possible, using the muscles in the area immediately above the knee.
      Note: This can also be accomplished by keeping the legs on the bed and lifting the heel off the bed slightly using the leg muscles.

IV. The patient states that the reason for coughing and deep breathing exercises is to keep the lungs well expanded and prevent congestion and demonstrates proper coughing and deep breathing techniques.

  A. Deep breathing
    1. If possible, this should be done in semi-Fowler's position.
    2. Rest the hands on the front or side of the midabdominal region so that expansion may be felt as breaths are taken.
    3. Breathe as deeply as possible through the nose and hold for a count of 5.
    4. Exhale through pursed lips, as though blowing out a candle.
    5. Do this 10 times every 1 to 2 hours.

	Content/ Reinforcement Delivered Date & RN	Learner Objectives Met Date & RN	Not Applicable

B. Coughing
  1. Take a few deep breaths.
  2. At the height of a deep breath, hack sharply 3 times.
  3. Breathe deeply again and cough strongly once or twice.
  4. Do this 3 times every 1 to 2 hours.
V. The patient describes the reasons for adequate fluid intake and states how much fluid should be consumed in a 24-hour period.
  A. The intake of fluids is designed to counteract losses from various sources such as urine and perspiration. Adequate fluid intake helps maintain a consistent urine output and contributes to the prevention of urinary complications.
  B. "The amount of fluid I should take each day is _____ glasses."
  C. Each time a full paper cup of fluid or any other volume of liquid is consumed, the amount should be reported to the nurse.
VI. The patient describes why position change is essential and how frequently it should be done.
  A. Position change is important because
    1. Prolonged pressure on any one area of the body restricts circulation to that area.
    2. Pressure leads to skin breakdown, which is uncomfortable and dangerous for the patient.
    3. Altering the position on a regular basis allows the circulation to be restored and promotes healthy skin.
    4. Position change is important for proper lung function.
  B. Position should be changed every 2 hours or more frequently if losses of sensation or fatigue occurs in any area.
VII. The patient describes symptoms that should be reported to the nurse immediately:
  A. Calf pain or tenderness
  B. Feeling of fatigue, numbness, or stinging in any area
  C. Pain or tightness in the chest
  D. Constipation
  E. Burning on urination; a feeling that the bladder is not completely emptied
VIII. The patient states why elastic stockings are necessary while immobilized and how often they should be removed.
  A. Elastic stockings are necessary to prevent pooling of blood in the lower extremities which can cause thrombophlebitis.
  B. Elastic stockings are removed for skin care twice daily.			

	Content/ Reinforcement Delivered Date & RN	Learner Objectives Met Date & RN	Not Applicable
Evaluation If patient or significant others are unable to complete some or all of this teaching plan, document evaluation in progress notes.			

	Content/ Reinforcement Delivered Date & RN	Learner Objectives Met Date & RN	Not Applicable

SURGICAL TREATMENT OF A FRACTURED HIP

Purpose

To diminish preoperative anxiety.
To familiarize the patient with postoperative care and to assess patient expectations.

Content

    I. Anatomy of the hip joint
   II. Brief discussion of the surgical procedure
  III. Review of the preoperative teaching plan
  IV. Routine before surgery
    V. Routine after surgery
  VI. Activity after discharge
 VII. Reasons to contact the physician
VIII. Follow-up

Learner Objectives

  I. The patient describes the anatomy of the hip joint.
    A. The hip is a ball and socket joint that allows free motion.
    B. The smooth rounded head of the thighbone (femur) fits into the deeply recessed socket (acetabulum) of the hip joint.
    C. The joint is covered by a tough, flexible protective capsule and is heavily reinforced by strong ligaments that stretch across the joint.
 II. The patient briefly discusses the surgical procedure.
    A. Moore's Arthroplasty. (See Figure 4.)
      1. This is treatment for a fracture of the head of the femur.
      2. An attempt is made to recreate a near normal hip.
      3. A prosthesis is inserted to replace the head of the femur and secured in place with bone cement.
      4. The fractured part is removed.
    B. Open reduction and internal fixation.
      1. This is usual treatment for a fractured hip.
      2. The hip is opened to provide visualization of the injury.
      3. The fracture is fixed with pins, nails, screws, plates, or a prosthesis (see Moore's arthroplasty).
III. The patient meets the objectives of the preoperative teaching plan.

	Content/ Reinforcement Delivered Date & RN	Learner Objectives Met Date & RN	Not Applicable

IV. The patient describes the routine on the day before surgery.
  A. Skin preparation
    1. A formal prep and shave are done in the operating room.
  B. Positioning
    1. The leg is immobilized in balanced suspension with Buck's traction.
    2. Balanced suspension is achieved by suspending the leg on a splint or frame to maintain alignment of the affected leg and to protect the leg from gravity.
    3. Buck's traction is achieved by attaching straps and a footplate to the lower leg, using ace bandages. Weights are added to the footplate to maintain alignment and reduce spasms that often accompany a fractured hip.
 	
V. The patient describes the routine after surgery.
  A. Intravenous (IV) and nutritional therapy.
    1. Intravenous therapy is necessary for the first few days after surgery as a means of fluid replacement.
    2. The patient is allowed nothing by mouth until fully awake. The diet is advanced slowly from liquids to a regular diet.
    3. IV fluids are continued until bowel sounds are present and the diet is tolerated.
    4. IV antibiotics are used for 48 hours postoperatively to prevent infection.
    5. Blood transfusions may be required during the immediate postoperative period to replace blood loss from surgery.
  B. Suction drainage
    1. The apparatus consists of a round container with a bulb on the end of it.
    2. A tube or drain that was inserted near the incision line during surgery is connected to the container to drain accumulating blood and fluids.
    3. The drain is kept in place 24 to 48 hours.
    4. Slight discomfort may be felt when the drains are removed.
  C. Positioning
    1. A pillow is kept between the legs to keep them apart.
    2. Turning is permitted only onto the affected hip with a pillow between the legs.
    3. The patient changes position in bed every 2 hours by holding onto the trapeze with the arms and pushing up off the bed with the unaffected leg.		

	Content/ Reinforcement Delivered Date & RN	Learner Objectives Met Date & RN	Not Applicable

4. When out of bed, the patient must sit in a high chair. The toilet must have a raised seat.
5. The foot of the affected leg must be kept in a neutral position.
D. Balanced suspension with Buck's traction
  1. Buck's traction is maintained for 48 to 72 hours after surgery.
  2. A footrest replaces the footplate when Buck's traction is discontinued. It prevents foot drop and facilitates ankle exercises.
  3. Balanced suspension is maintained for 7 to 10 days after surgery and then only at night.
E. Ambulation
  1. Instruction is given by the nurse or physical therapist.
  2. Activities include transfer from bed to chair on the first to third postoperative day or may be delayed if the fracture is unstable.
  3. Gait training is taught by the nurse or physical therapist, and the patient progresses from walker to crutches.
  4. Ambulation begins on the second to third postoperative day and weight bearing is limited to touchdown.
VI. The patient describes activity after discharge.
VII. The patient describes the reasons to contact the physician
 	
A. Increased hip pain
B. Changes in color, sensation, or movement
  1. Dusky or pale color of the foot of the affected leg
  2. Cool or very hot feelings in the foot
  3. Decreased sensation in the foot, numbness, or tingling
  4. Decreased movement of the foot or leg
C. An inability to move the affected leg freely toward the midline
VIII. The patient states the date and time of follow-up appointment and the following phone numbers:
Follow-up appointment: _____
Physician #: _____
Orthopedic clinic #: _____
Emergency room #: _____			

	Content/ Reinforcement Delivered Date & RN	Learner Objectives Met Date & RN	Not Applicable
Evaluation If patient or significant others are unable to complete some or all of this teaching plan, document evaluation in progress notes.			

Figure 4 Moore's Arthroplasty

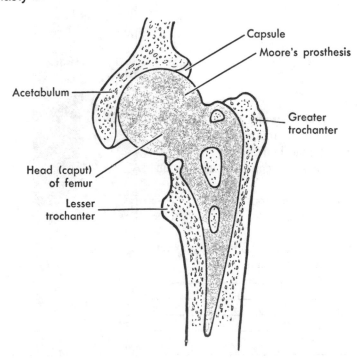

	Content/ Reinforcement Delivered Date & RN	Learner Objectives Met Date & RN	Not Applicable

UNNA BOOT

Purpose

To provide the patient with information regarding the use of the Unna boot.

Content

    I. Etiology of venous ulcer
   II. Unna boot and its function
  III. Routine checkup
  IV. Reasons to contact physician
    V. Home care
  VI. Handout
 VII. Follow-up

Learner Objectives

    I. Patient states etiology of venous ulcers.
      A. Venous ulcers are a result of a pooling of blood in the lower extremities. The veins are unable to maintain adequate blood flow to the skin surface, which causes a breakdown in the skin and can progress deeper into the tissue surface. Impaired blood flow can be caused by the following conditions:
        1. Diabetes mellitus
        2. Arteriosclerosis with venous insufficiency
        3. Trauma aggravated by poor wound healing
        4. Phlebitis
        5. Obesity
   II. Patient describes an Unna boot and its functions.
      A. The Unna boot is a gauze bandage coated with calamine lotion. The application of the boot from ankle to knee, literally covering the area of ulcer, will provide two functions:
        1. Protection of the ulcer and the skin surrounding the ulcer
        2. Application of pressure to the veins of the legs promoting increased venous return, which is necessary for increased circulation and healing of the ulcer
  III. Patient describes routine checkup.
      A. The boot must be changed at least once a week.
      B. In cases where the ulcer is deep and draining through the boot and covers the dressing, it may have to be changed two to three times a week for 2 to 3 weeks or until the drainage subsides.

	Content/ Reinforcement Delivered Date & RN	Learner Objectives Met Date & RN	Not Applicable

C. When the boot is removed, the ulcer is measured and the type and character of drainage is recorded.
D. The entire leg is then washed thoroughly with phisohex and dried with a towel.
E. Another boot is applied.
IV. Patient states reasons to contact physician or nurse.
  A. The patient will return to the clinic or emergency room if the following problems develop:
    1. Pain or aching sensation in the legs or feet
    2. Change in color of the toes
    3. Numbness or tingling of the toes
    4. Disturbance in integrity of the boot
    5. Damage to the boot because of inadvertent moisture as a result of showering, rain, etc.
V. Patient describes home care of the boot.
  A. The boot is not to be removed. (Removing the boot may cause more skin damage.)
  B. If there are problems with the boot, the patient can come to the emergency room at any time and to the physician's office during operating hours.
  C. The boot should not get wet. The patient should avoid showers or baths and exposure to the elements (rain, snow, etc.).
VI. The patient takes the handout home.
VII. Patient describes follow-up:
  A. Appointment with
    Physician: _____
  B. How to contact physician
    Physician #: _____
    Emergency room #: _____
 	
Evaluation
 	
If patient or significant others are unable to complete some or all of the teaching plan, document evaluation in progress notes.			

PATIENT HANDOUT FOR UNNA BOOT

I. *What is an ulcer?*

An ulcer is a result of poor circulation. The blood "pools" in certain areas of the leg and does not provide adequate nutrition to the skin, which leads to a breakdown in the skin surface, which leads to ulcer formation.

II. *How is your ulcer treated?*

The ulcer is treated with applications of an Unna boot, which is a gauze bandage coated with calamine lotion. The boot heals the ulcer in two ways: (1) it acts as a protective skin covering and (2) it compresses the veins to the area thus promoting good blood flow to the ulcer which is essential for wound healing.

III. *What are important observations to make?*

The boot can cause some constriction of the vessels of the leg, resulting in

1. Pain or aching sensation in legs or feet
2. Change in color of toes
3. Numbness or tingling of toes
4. Disturbance in integrity of boot
5. Damage to boot because of inadvertent moisture as a result of showering, rain, etc.

   If any are noted, please contact physician or nurse immediately.

IV. *How often should you return?*

The boot must be changed at least weekly and, in cases of increased draining, two to three times a week.

V. *How should you care for an Unna boot?*

You should not attempt to remove the boot. You should avoid any moisture to boot. This means avoiding showers, baths, and exposure to the elements (rain, snow, etc.).

VI. *Can I resume all my daily activities?*

Yes, however, if you elevate your legs for 3 to 4 hours during the day, the ulcer will heal at a more rapid rate.

Part VI

The Neurological System

	Content/ Reinforcement Delivered Date & RN	Learner Objectives Met Date & RN	Not Applicable

SEIZURE

Purpose

To teach the patient or significant other the characteristics of a seizure disorder and its management at home.

Content

I. Definition of a seizure
II. Description of characteristics of the patient's seizure
III. Management of the patient during and after a seizure
IV. Anticonvulsant medications
V. Safety measures at home
VI. Reasons to notify the physician
VII. Follow-up

Learner Objectives

I. Patient and significant other describe a seizure in simple terms and identify the specific seizure disorder.
   A. A seizure is a symptom of a disturbance of nervous system function that may be caused by trauma, infection, fever, metabolic disorder, drug intoxication, or unknown cause.
   B. The seizure disorder is:
      1. Grand mal
      2. Petit mal
      3. Febrile
      4. Abstinence
      5. Focal
      6. Other _____
II. Patient and significant other describe the characteristics of patient's type of seizure:
   A. Loss of consciousness
   B. Body twitching
   C. Aura
   D. Incontinence
   E. Eyes deviated to side
   F. Staring spells
   G. Vomiting or foaming at mouth
   H. Incoherence
   I. Postictal stage
   J. Other _____
III. Patient or significant other states management during seizure activity.
   A. Remain with patient during seizure.

	Content/ Reinforcement Delivered Date & RN	Learner Objectives Met Date & RN	Not Applicable

B. Observe duration and describe seizure.
C. Do not try to stop the seizure by slapping the face or giving medications.
D. Do not physically restrain the patient.
E. Protect the patient from self-injury by turning the head and the body to the side and place a soft object under the head.
F. Do not put hard objects into the mouth. The patient will not "swallow" the tongue when the head is turned to the side.
G. If the patient is turning blue, clear the airway and give mouth-to-mouth breathing.
H. During postictal state, patient will be tired and may complain of headache, restlessness, or muscle weakness.
I. Other _____
IV. Patient or significant other describes anticonvulsant medication and meets objectives of the medication teaching guide.
V. Patient or significant other states safety measures.
  A. If a child, do not leave the patient unattended in a high chair.
  B. If the patient is a child, keep bed and play area free of hard objects to protect the child from harm.
  C. Activity is not restricted but caution should be taken in high areas, during gymnastics, in work area, and while swimming.
  D. Patient is to wear medic alert identification.
  E. Work and school nurse should know of patient's seizure disorder.
  F. If the patient has an aura, the patient should seek privacy and a safe place to lie down before the seizure.
  G. Automobile licensure is regulated by states. Inquire about the rules for the seizure patient through the registry of motor vehicles.
  H. The work environment should be evaluated for safety, e.g., high construction area.
VI. The patient or significant other states when to contact physician.
  A. Seizure activity persists or there is increased frequency.
  B. The patient is unable to take medication.
  C. Other _____
VII. The patient or significant other describes follow-up care.
  A. Keep a record of seizures, noting date, time, description of seizures.
  B. Support system is available through epilepsy society.			

	Content/ Reinforcement Delivered Date & RN	Learner Objectives Met Date & RN	Not Applicable
C. Follow-up appointment ——————— D. Physician #: —————————— Emergency room #: ———————			

Evaluation

If patient or significant others are unable to complete some or all of this teaching plan, document evaluation in progress notes.

	Content/ Reinforcement Delivered Date & RN	Learner Objectives Met Date & RN	Not Applicable
HEAD TRAUMA			

HEAD TRAUMA

Purpose

To familiarize the patient or significant other with the nature of the injury.

To familiarize the patient or significant other with the possible complications that may arise from the head injury and that would necessitate medical attention.

To provide patient or significant other with instructions for follow-up care.

Content

  I. Anatomy of the head
  II. Normal and abnormal events that may occur after a head injury
  III. Additional reasons to contact the physician
  IV. Instructions for follow-up care
  V. Patient handout

Learner Objectives

  I. The patient or significant other describes the basic anatomy of the head:
    A. The skull is the bony outer covering of the head.
    B. The dura is a tough membranous covering beneath the skull.
    C. Blood vessels, located beneath the dura, help supply oxygen to the brain.
    D. Cerebrospinal fluid surrounds and cushions the brain.

  II. The patient or significant other describes the difference between the normal events following a head injury and the abnormal events that would necessitate contacting a physician:
    A. Swelling
      1. Normal Events
        a) Observe the extent and nature of the swelling currently present.
        b) Ice should be applied to constrict the blood vessels and decrease swelling.
      2. Abnormal Events
        a) The physician should be notified for a large soft lump not previously noted. This new swelling may be at the area of the head injury or in a different area.

	Content/ Reinforcement Delivered Date & RN	Learner Objectives Met Date & RN	Not Applicable

B. Drowsiness
  1. Normal Events
    a) The patient may be more tired after the head injury. The patient may go to sleep at the normal bedtime, but if the injury occurred in the evening, he should be awakened every 2 hours throughout the night to check alertness.
  2. Abnormal Events
    a) The physician should be notified if it is difficult to arouse the patient.
C. Vomiting
  1. Normal Events
    a) The patient may vomit once or twice after the head injury.
  2. Abnormal Events
    a) The physician should be notified for persistent projectile vomiting.
D. Headaches
  1. Normal Events
    a) Mild headache, which can be relieved by use of Tylenol, is normal.
  2. Abnormal Events
    a) The physician should be notified for continued or severe headache that is not relieved by Tylenol.
 	
III. The physician should also be notified if any of the following events are observed:
 	
A. Seizures evidenced by trembling, jerking, or shaking of any body part; fainting or loss of consciousness
B. Clumsy walking, which may be evidenced by favoring one leg or loss of balance while walking
C. Unequal pupils in which the pupil of one eye is larger than the other
D. Weakness of body limbs, evidenced by favoring or weakness of one side of the body or numbness or tingling of arms or legs
E. Difficulty speaking normally, mumbling, thick speech, or inability to speak
 	
IV. Follow-up care
A. The patient or significant other states local care of site of injury, i.e., laceration care if sutures are required.
B. The patient or significant other states how to contact physician if abnormal complications occur.
    Physician #: _____
 	
V. The patient or significant other takes home head injury instruction handout			

	Content/ Reinforcement Delivered Date & RN	Learner Objectives Met Date & RN	Not Applicable
Evaluation If patient or significant others are unable to complete some or all of this teaching plan, document evaluation in progress notes.			

	Content/ Reinforcement Delivered Date & RN	Learner Objectives Met Date & RN	Not Applicable

CRANIOTOMY

Purpose

To help the patient understand the surgical procedure and its complications.
To ensure understanding and participation in preoperative and postoperative care.

Content

    I. Anatomy and physiology of brain and aims for surgery
   II. Preoperative events
  III. Routines the day before and the morning of surgery
  IV. Respiratory care
   V. Issues related to safety
  VI. Events related to recovery
 VII. Reasons to contact the physician
VIII. Restrictions on activity after discharge
  IX. Discharge medication
   X. Performance of activities of daily living (ADLs)
  XI. Support services at home
 XII. Follow-up after discharge

Learner Objectives

  I. The patient describes in simple terms the anatomy and physiology of the brain and the aims for surgery.
    A. The patient's anomaly, disease, or injury

    B. Surgical procedures to be performed

    C. Expected outcomes

	Content/ Reinforcement Delivered Date & RN	Learner Objectives Met Date & RN	Not Applicable

II. The patient describes in general terms the preop events.
  A. Diagnostic tests
    1. Blood tests, urine specimens, and EKG are done to help assess health prior to surgery.
    2. A chest x-ray is taken to assess the respiratory status.
    3. A CAT scan, a computerized x-ray, shows structural changes in the skull and brain. It also shows the location of abnormalities.
    4. Angiography (for patients with vascular problems) locates and assesses the condition of blood vessels prior to surgery. Dye is injected into the blood vessels and x-rays are taken.
    5. A neuro-assessment is done prior to surgery. It helps determine location of the lesion and establishes a baseline for comparison after surgery.
 	
  B. Routines the day before and the morning of surgery
    1. The surgeon or one of his assistants will explain the surgery and ask that a legal consent for surgery be signed.
    2. The patient's hair is washed with an antimicrobial solution two or three times as an added protection against infection.
    3. Smoking is discouraged to decrease the risk of postoperative respiratory complications.
    4. Nothing is consumed by mouth after midnight because the stomach must be empty to prevent nausea or vomiting during the operation.
    5. Ace wraps or thigh high stockings are applied to help improve circulation, because the patient will be motionless for many hours during surgery.
    6. Intramuscular medication is given to induce drowsiness and relaxation.
    7. Transportation to the operating room is provided on a stretcher.
    8. Intravenous lines will be started.
    9. Staff will be wearing face masks and hair covering.
    10. In the operating room the patient's hair will be shaved and the head scrubbed with antiseptic solution. The patient is usually "put to sleep" before this is started.
    11. A special tube is inserted through the nose or mouth to assist with breathing. A sore throat may be experienced postoperatively due to this tube.			

	Content/ Reinforcement Delivered Date & RN	Learner Objectives Met Date & RN	Not Applicable

III. The patient describes in general terms what can be expected postoperatively.
 	
A. Recovery room
    1. When surgery is complete, the patient is immediately brought to the recovery room where nurses and doctors will be watching closely.
    2. The recovery room is usually a busy, noisy area.
    3. The patient may wake up in the recovery room but will often be very drowsy.
    4. Patients rarely remember being in the recovery room.
 	
B. Postoperative equipment patient may encounter
    1. The endotracheal tube is used to assist breathing. It is not possible to talk while the tube is in place because it goes through the voice box. It may be removed by the time the patient awakens or it may remain in place for a few hours or until the next morning.
    2. The nasogastric tube is a small tube that is inserted through the nose, connecting with the back of the throat and down into the stomach. It prevents nausea and vomiting and may be used for giving medications. It will probably be removed the next morning or when bowel sounds return.
    3. Intravenous and arterial lines for medications and fluid maintenance are in place. An arterial line is used to draw blood and to monitor blood pressure.
    4. A Foley catheter for drainage is generally in place until the next morning. The urge to void is caused by feeling the catheter against the bladder neck.
    5. One or more drains are placed to drain blood and fluid from the surgical site and to promote healing.
    6. Depending on the location of the surgical site a dressing may cover the neck or part or all of the head. It frequently feels tight.
    7. Continuous EKG monitoring is maintained while in the recovery room and ICU-5. The arterial line may be connected to a monitor for a continuous reading of blood pressure.
 	
C. Treatments and procedures in the intensive care unit
    1. Blood pressure, temperature, pulse, respiratory rate, and the neuro-assessment are done every one half to two hours for the first postoperative day. Nurses and doctors will repeatedly ask simple questions and request that simple things be demonstrated (e.g., sticking out the tongue, squeezing hands).			

	Content/ Reinforcement Delivered	Learner Objectives Met	Not Applicable
	Date & RN	Date & RN	

    2. Fluids are closely monitored. An accurate urine output is kept.

    3. The nurse will frequently check drains and dressings for the amount and type of drainage from incisional wounds. Most drains will be removed the second or third postop day.

    4. Pain medication is not routinely given after a craniotomy. This is because the staff must evaluate the patient's level of consciousness and orientation.

    5. The morning after surgery, activity is increased. The patient will be encouraged to do as much as possible.

    6. Fluids and a progressive diet are encouraged when the patient is fully awake and anesthesia has completely worn off.

  D. Symptoms following a craniotomy that the patient should report to the nurse

    1. Headache

    2. Dizziness

    3. Extremity weakness or sensory change

    4. Speech difficulties

    5. Thirst

    6. Lethargy

    7. Swallowing difficulties

IV. The patient identifies respiratory care following surgery.

  A. Some patients may remain intubated for a while following surgery to help clear secretions. It is impossible to talk with the endotracheal tube in place. The ability to talk will return when the tube is removed.

  B. An oxygen face mask provides oxygen and humidification.

  C. Coughing and deep breathing are encouraged to expand and clear the lungs of secretions.

  D. The patient may use an incentive spirometer to help keep his lungs expanded.

  E. Respiratory care may include chest physical therapy. The nurse will slap the patient's back fairly vigorously in order to help loosen secretions and help the patient to breathe deeply. This treatment helps to produce a good, productive cough.

V. The patient identifies issues related to safety and how to prevent slips and falls.

  A. Call the nurse for assistance to the bathroom.

  B. Sit and stand up slowly.

  C. If confused, safety restraints may be used.

	Content/ Reinforcement Delivered Date & RN	Learner Objectives Met Date & RN	Not Applicable

VI. The patient describes normal events related to recovery.
   A. Activity is gradually increased as motor function and strength develop.
   B. Assistance is given to help the patient gradually increase abilities to feed, bathe, and dress himself.
   C. Bladder function may return slowly. If unable to void, a catheter will be used to assist with elimination.
   D. Energy and muscle strength will gradually increase with physical therapy and time.
VII. Patient describes reasons to contact the physician after discharge.
   A. A temperature above 99°F.
   B. Redness, pain, or drainage around the surgical incision
   C. Recurrent headaches
   D. Seizures
   E. Dizziness or fainting
   F. Fall with injury to the head
VIII. Patient describes activity restrictions after discharge.
   A. No heavy lifting or vigorous activity.
   B. For six months after surgery an automobile vehicle should not be driven.
IX. The patient meets the objectives of the medication treatment plan for the following discharge medications.
   A. _____
   B. _____
   C. _____
   D. _____
X. The patient describes how activities of daily living will be performed.
   A. Obtain and prepare food
 	
   B. Adapt living conditions
 	
   C Obtain transportation			

	Content/ Reinforcement Delivered Date & RN	Learner Objectives Met Date & RN	Not Applicable
D. Ensure self-care			
XI. The patient identifies support services in the community that will provide assistance at home. 　　1. The family or a significant other			
2. Other			
XII. The patient identifies follow-up appointments and how to contact the physician. Physician Appointment			
Physician #: _____ Emergency room #: _____ Other Appointment			

Part VII

The Female Reproductive System

	Content/ Reinforcement Delivered	Learner Objectives Met	Not Applicable
	Date & RN	Date & RN	

BREAST SELF-EXAM

Purpose

To ensure the patient's ability to independently perform breast self-examination.

Content

  I. The importance of breast self-exam
 II. The visual and physical exam
III. Familial influences and medications
 IV. Reasons to contact the physician or nurse
  V. Distribution of handout
 VI. Follow-up care

Learner Objectives

  I. The patient states the reason for breast self-exam.
     A. Breast self-exam enables early detection of breast changes.
 II. The patient describes and demonstrates when and how to do a physical exam:
     A. Time of the procedure
        1. Examine the breast at the same time each month, on the day following a period or, if menopausal, choose a date and do the exam on this date each month.
     B. Visual exam
        1. Perform the exam while standing or sitting in front of a mirror.
           a) Arms at side, observe.
           b) Hands placed on top of head, bring elbows back.
           c) Hands on hips, squeeze, bring shoulders forward.
        2. Look for any changes in the breast or nipple contour.
           a) Any prominent lumps
           b) Nipple discharge
           c) Dimpling
           d) Unusual puckering
           e) Inversion of nipple
           f) Discoloration of breast
     C. Physical exam
        1. Place the right arm on top of the head for examination of the right breast and vice versa for the left breast.

	Content/ Reinforcement Delivered Date & RN	Learner Objectives Met Date & RN	Not Applicable
2. Use the left hand for exam of the right breast. Use the right hand for exam of the left breast. 3. Use the whole hand, palms with fingers flat, tucking the thumb under palm, fingers held together. 4. The hand compresses firmly yet gently against the chest wall while moving in a circular motion. 5. A systematic approach to the breast exam begins at 12:00, moves clockwise, firmly but gently. Palpate breast starting from the outer limit to the nipple. 6. The fingers remain on the skin when moving to the next area. 7. Palpate the entire breast then squeeze the nipple horizontally and vertically to note any discharge. 8. Feel under the arm. The patient may be encouraged to perform breast self-exam in the shower or tub. Cover the breast with soap; this enables the hand to slide more easily and the touch is more sensitive. III. The patient describes familial influences and medications that may contribute to breast disease: A. Previous history of breast disease in the family B. Use of birth control pills C. Use of DES (diethylstilbestrol) during mother's pregnancy IV. The patient states that she will contact the physician or nurse immediately with any unusual findings noted on breast self-exam. V. The patient takes a handout on breast self-exam home. VI. Follow-up A. The patient states that she does breast exam monthly. B. The patient performs an adequate examination by review.			
Evaluation If patient or significant others are unable to complete some or all of this teaching plan, document evaluation in progress notes.			

	Content/ Reinforcement Delivered Date & RN	Learner Objectives Met Date & RN	Not Applicable

DIAPHRAGM

Purpose

To enable the patient to correctly use the diaphragm as a method of birth control.

Content

    I. Female reproductive anatomy and physiology
   II. Types of diaphragms
  III. The diaphragm as a method of birth control
  IV. Diaphragm fitting
   V. Insertion and removal of the diaphragm
  VI. Proper use of the diaphragm
 VII. Distribution of handout

Learner Objectives

    I. Patient describes the female reproductive anatomy and physiology.
       A. The normal female anatomy consists of vagina, cervix, uterus, Fallopian tubes, and ovaries. Eggs (ova) are produced in the ovaries. Midway during the menstrual cycle, the eggs are released (ovulation) into the pelvic cavity and travel into the Fallopian tubes.
       B. During intercourse, sperm are deposited into the vagina. They travel through the cervix into the uterus and then to the Fallopian tubes.
       C. Fertilization (union of sperm and ovum) takes place in the Fallopian tubes. The fertilized ovum travels to the uterus for implantation. If fertilization does not take place, menstruation occurs.
   II. Patient identifies her type of diaphragm:
       A. Arching spring
       B. Coil spring
       C. Flat spring
  III. Patient describes how the diaphragm works as a method of birth control.
       A. The diaphragm acts as a mechanical barrier, covering the cervical os (opening).
       B. The cervix is covered by the rubber dome of the diaphragm, which holds spermicidal jelly or cream against cervical os.
  IV. Patient describes the proper size and fit of diaphragm.
       A. The size is determined by the health care provider.
       B. The diaphragm should be refitted if there is a greater than 20-pound weight gain, after a delivery or pelvic surgery, and at the annual exam.

	Content/ Reinforcement Delivered Date & RN	Learner Objectives Met Date & RN	Not Applicable

V. Patient inserts and removes diaphragm.
   A. Patient checks the proper placement over the cervix by feeling the cervix through the dome and feeling the rim of the diaphragm behind the pubic bone.
   B. Proper fit is then checked by the nurse.
VI. Patient describes the basic principles of using the diaphragm, cream or jelly, and applicator.
   A. Use 1 tablespoon of spermicidal cream or jelly in dome of diaphragm before initial insertion.
   B. The diaphragm may be inserted up to 2 hours before intercourse and must be left in place 6 to 8 hours after intercourse.
   C. The diaphragm should not be left in place for more than 24 hours.
   D. An applicator full of cream or jelly must be used with each subsequent act of intercourse, being careful not to remove the diaphragm. You must leave the diaphragm in another 6 to 8 hours from the time of last intercourse.
   E. After removing the diaphragm, wash with mild soap and water, and dry thoroughly before storing in plastic case.
   F. Before using the diaphragm, check for tears, holes, and signs of wear by holding it up to light.
   G. Do not use Vaseline, powder, or cornstarch on diaphragm at any time.
   H. The diaphragm should be used at all times, even during the menstrual period.
VII. The patient takes a handout on the diaphragm.
 	
Evaluation
 	
If the patient or significant others are unable to complete some or all of this teaching plan, document evaluation in progress notes.			

	Content/ Reinforcement Delivered Date & RN	Learner Objectives Met Date & RN	Not Applicable

PREOPERATIVE AND POSTOPERATIVE DILATATION AND CURETTAGE

Purpose

To teach the patient about the preoperative, postoperative, and at-home routine associated with a dilatation and curettage (D&C).

Content

   I. Anatomy related to dilatation and curettage
  II. Definition of dilatation and curettage
 III. Routine before procedure
 IV. Description of procedure
  V. Routine after procedure
 VI. Care at home
VII. Contacting the physician
VIII. Follow-up

Learner Objectives

  I. The patient describes the pertinent anatomy of the reproductive tract.
    A. Uterus
      1. Fundus
      2. Cervix
      3. Os
    B. Vagina
 II. The patient defines a D&C as:
    A. Dilatation of the opening of the uterus (os)
    B. A scraping (curettage) of the lining of the uterus (endometrium)
    C. The reason for having a D&C is:

    _____

    _____

III. The patient describes the routine before a D&C.
    A. Nothing by mouth is allowed after midnight.
    B. Cigarette smoking is to be avoided for at least 24 hours before surgery.
    C. Pre-op blood work is done.
    D. An operation permit is signed.
    E. Intravenous therapy is started to ensure proper hydration.
    F. The skin is washed with an antiseptic soap.
    G. A sedative is given before transportation to the operating room.

	Content/ Reinforcement Delivered	Learner Objectives Met	Not Applicable
	Date & RN	Date & RN	
IV. The patient describes the events of the procedure. A. The patient is placed in stirrups. B. Local anesthesia (Xylocaine) is given. C. Some uterine cramping is experienced as the os is opened and the endometrium is scraped. D. When the procedure is over a peripad is put in place and the patient is transported to the recovery room. V. The patient states the postoperative procedure as follows: A. Vital signs will be taken frequently. B. The peripad will be checked for bleeding. C. When sufficiently awake and ambulatory, the patient may go home. D. Someone should be available to accompany the patient home. VI. The patient describes what to do and what to expect at home. A. There will be period-like bleeding for 2–3 days, followed by spotting and staining that may last for 2 weeks. B. There may be mild uterine cramping for 24–48 hours. This should be relieved with a mild analgesic. C. Peripads should be used rather than tampons. D. Do not douche. E. No vaginal intercourse for two weeks. VII. The patient states she will contact the physician for any of the following reasons: A. Heavy bleeding with or without clots. B. Temperature above 99°F. C. Abdominal pain. D. Other concerns or problems. Physician # _____ Emergency room # _____ VIII. The patient states the date and time of her follow-up appointment. _____			

Evaluation

If patient or significant others are unable to complete some or all of this teaching plan, document evaluation in progress notes.

	Content/ Reinforcement Delivered Date & RN	Learner Objectives Met Date & RN	Not Applicable

MASTECTOMY

Purpose

To facilitate the physical and psychological adjustment of the patient undergoing mastectomy or axillary lymph node dissection for breast cancer.

Content

    I. Preoperative procedures
   II. Postoperative procedures
  III. Reach to Recovery visit
  IV. Breast prosthesis
   V. Arm and shoulder exercises
  VI. Incision care
 VII. Hand and arm care
VIII. Postoperative activity levels: limits and goals
  IX. Breast self-exam teaching plan
   X. Psychological needs and support systems
  XI. Discharge planning
 XII. Signs and symptoms of recurrence

Learner Objectives

  I. Patient describes preoperative events and rationale for surgery.
    A. The patient describes events during the day before surgery.
       1. A physical exam and blood work are performed.
       2. Nothing is allowed by mouth after midnight.
       3. The incision area may be washed and shaved.
       4. Medications are given to cause drowsiness and relaxation. The mouth will be dry.
    B. The patient describes the type of surgery to be performed:
       1. Radical mastectomy: removal of the breast, axillary nodes, and pectoralis muscle
       2. Modified radical mastectomy: removal of the breast and axillary nodes
       3. Simple mastectomy: removal of breast tissues only
    C. The patient describes the rationale for surgery:
       1. To remove cancerous tissue from the breast
       2. To examine axillary nodes for possible metastases and aid in treatment planning

| | Content/ Reinforcement Delivered

Date & RN | Learner Objectives Met

Date & RN | Not Applicable |
|---|---|---|---|
| D. The patient describes the initial postoperative appearance of the chest wall.
　1. The chest wall will be flat.
　2. A horizontal incision will be made whenever possible (check with physician).
　3. The incision will be covered by a dressing.
　4. There will be drainage tubes from the surgical site to a container (called a *Davol* or *Hemovac*).
　5. The incisional area may be red and swollen.

II. The patient describes postoperative events.
　A. Wake-up will be in the recovery room.
　　1. Frequent vital signs are taken
　　2. Oxygen is administered
　　3. IV fluids are administered
　　4. EKG leads are attached
　B. Pain medication is available.
　C. Deep breathing, coughing, and use of blow bottles are encouraged to clear the lungs.
　D. The affected arm and hand are positioned with a sling or pillows.
　E. Common postop physical sensations include
　　1. Nausea and vomiting
　　2. Discomfort at the incision sites (for which medication is available)
　　3. Tightness, pulling at the incision sites causing limited range of motion of the arm and shoulder
　　4. Numbness at the incision sites
　　5. "Pins and needles" or brief, sharp twinges near the incision site or underarm
　　6. A general sense of tiredness or low energy
The patient states that these are usually temporary and will diminish with time. There is a great deal of variation and response to sensation with individual patients.

III. The patient describes the goals and services of Reach to Recovery volunteers and how to arrange a visit with the physician's approval:
　A. Goals: "To assist patient to achieve her maximum potential emotionally, physically and socially"
　B. Services
　　1. Provides an opportunity to visit with another woman who has undergone breast cancer surgery
　　2. Provides brochures that
　　　a) Discuss postsurgical emotional adjustment
　　　b) Describe arm exercises
　　　c) List establishments where prostheses, bras, and bathing suits can be purchased | | | |

	Content/ Reinforcement Delivered Date & RN	Learner Objectives Met Date & RN	Not Applicable
3. Provides a free "temporary" breast prosthesis (a soft, lightweight fiber-filled form) to be worn home from the hospital			
IV. The patient describes when and how to obtain a breast prosthesis.			
A. If a Reach to Recovery volunteer cannot visit the patient before discharge, arrangements for obtaining temporary prostheses can be made by			
1. Calling the American Cancer Society and arranging for a family member to stop by and pick up the prosthesis (free)			
2. Calling the nurse to assist in scheduling a visit from a professional fitter			
3. Directing a family member to an intimate apparel shop or medical supply company where a prosthesis can be purchased (cost: $6 to 10)			
B. The patient demonstrates how to fasten the temporary prosthesis into a bra and adjust the padding to match the size and shape of the opposite breast.			
C. The patient tries on the bra and prosthesis and clothes to be worn home and makes final aesthetic adjustments.			
D. The patient goes for a walk to "try it out," accompanied by a nurse or significant other.			
E. The patient states that she will ask the doctor at the first or second postoperative visit if her incision is healed sufficiently for a weighted breast prosthesis (permanent prosthesis) to be fitted. The patient will obtain a prescription in order to submit the cost of the prosthesis for insurance coverage. The patient states that she can obtain a list of trained fitters and companies that supply a large variety of styles. (A list is compiled by Reach to Recovery.)			
V. The patient contacts a physical therapist if ordered by the physician and demonstrates the following exercises when appropriate.			
A. Initial exercises per order of physician			
1. Chest expansion with hands placed on upper chest			
2. Arm rotation exercises with elbow bent to 90° and arm pressed against body			
3. Shoulder shrugs			
4. Hand squeezes, using a gauze roll			
B. Advanced exercises per order of physician			
1. Wall climbing			
2. Forward arm raises			
3. Rope pull			
4. Lateral arm raises against a wall			

	Content/ Reinforcement Delivered Date & RN	Learner Objectives Met Date & RN	Not Applicable
C. The patient states that she will continue exercises at home until full strength and range of motion return.			
VI. The patient describes incision care at home.			
A. Inspect the incision area before discharge to establish baseline criteria for observation of infection or complications.			
B. Keep the area clean and dry.			
C. Avoid pressure and constrictive clothing.			
D. (With physician's approval) may shower, avoiding direct spray, very hot water, harsh cleansers, and talcum powder on incision.			
E. Call physician promptly if the following occur:			
1. Increased redness or swelling			
2. Thick yellow drainage from incision			
3. Temperature over 100°F.			
4. Increased drainage or bleeding that soaks the dressing			
VII. The patient describes hand and arm care integral to the prevention of lymphedema. (*Note:* This does not apply to the patient who has had a simple mastectomy.)			
A. Defines *lymphedema* as swelling of affected arm due to accumulation of fluid secondary to the removal of the axillary lymph nodes.			
B. Describes possible causes of lymphedema in the affected arm:			
1. Trauma or injury			
2. Constrictive clothing, jewelry, or anything that inhibits circulation			
3. Alteration in skin integrity resulting in infection			
C. Describes ways to prevent lymphedema.			
1. Elevate arm at first sign of any swelling using gravity to reduce fluid accumulation.			
2. Offer unaffected arm for venipuncture, injection, and blood pressure.			
3. Use elbow length hot pad mits around stove and burners.			
4. Use mild soaps or wears rubber gloves if using harsh detergents or chemicals.			
5. Keep cuticles pushed back to prevent hangnails, tears.			
6. Use hand creams to keep skin and cuticles soft and intact.			
7. Treat all cuts and scratches immediately by washing with soap and water and applying mild antiseptic.			
8. Wear insect spray to avoid insect bites and stings.			
9. Avoid tight clothes, rings, and bracelets.			

	Content/ Reinforcement Delivered	Learner Objectives Met	Not Applicable
	Date & RN	Date & RN	

10. Use extra caution when shaving under arms to avoid nicks or will use a cream hair remover (first testing small area for sensitivity).

The patient states that these precautions will always be necessary.

D. Lists the signs and symptoms of lymphangitis and states that she will notify the physician immediately if they occur:
1. Swelling that does not decrease after a few days of elevation and rest
2. Swelling that is accompanied by tightness, redness in upper arm or chest area, and temperature over 100°F.
3. Sensation of pins in arm accompanied by preceding symptoms

VIII. The patient describes guidelines for resuming activities of daily living (ADL).
A. Initial postoperative limitations or restrictions.
1. Avoid strenuous activities and lifting of heavy objects until clearance is given by a physician.
2. Avoid fatigue by scheduling rest and recreational periods in her day as needed.
3. Carry packages and heavier objects on unaffected side.

B. Goals of recovery
1. To regain arm strength and range of motion gradually and steadily by performing prescribed exercises, light household tasks, and ADLs
2. To resume self-care activities, e.g., dressing, bathing, grooming
3. To promote complete tissue healing and return of energy level by eating well-balanced meals, high in protein, e.g., red meat, fish, poultry, tofu products, dairy products
4. To gain tolerance and patience for normal variation in daily levels of energy, range of motion, comfort, and mood

IX. The patient meets the objectives of the breast self-exam teaching plan (for remaining breast).

X. The patient lists common psychological hurdles or difficult events of rehabilitation process:
A. Waiting for final pathology report and discussion regarding need for additional therapy
B. Viewing incision for the first time and grieving for lost breast
C. Significant other or spouse viewing incision for the first time

	Content/ Reinforcement Delivered Date & RN	Learner Objectives Met Date & RN	Not Applicable
D. Resumption of physical and sexual intimacy E. Being fitted for and purchasing first weighted prosthesis F. Obtaining information regarding breast reconstruction and making a decision whether to have it done G. Resuming work, social contacts, and activities H. Seeking out and accepting outside support or therapy to help cope with the experience XI. The patient reviews discharge planning: A. Time and place of first postop exam Date: _____ Time: _____ Location: _____ Physician #: _____ B. Notification of physician regarding postoperative complications or concerns. Physician telephone #: _____ C. The patient meets the objectives of the medication teaching plan. D. If home care is set up (VNA, physical therapy, etc.) Agency phone #: _____ Date: _____			
XII. The patient describes signs and symptoms to observe between physician's exams: A. Any new lump, at mastectomy site, or in remaining breast B. Bone pain C. Persistent cough or hoarseness D. Unexplained weight loss E. A sore that does not heal The patient states that these are possible symptoms of recurrent disease, but that in vast majority of cases they are due to common conditions such as arthritis, flu or cold, irritations from environment, change in diet or sleep patterns. The patient will contact the physician if she detects a change or has a concern.			

Evaluation

If patient or significant others are unable to complete some or all of this teaching plan, document evaluation in progress notes.

	Content/ Reinforcement Delivered	Learner Objectives Met	Not Applicable
	Date & RN	Date & RN	

RADIUM INSERTION FOR GYNECOLOGY PATIENTS

Purpose

To ensure the patient's understanding of the therapy, daily routine, and protective measures associated with radium implantation.
To recognize and allow the patient to express her feelings about her disease and this procedure.

Content

    I. Description of hospital routine and policies relative to radium implant therapy
    II. Routine preoperative procedures
   III. Postoperative procedures
   IV. Policies regarding a dislodged radium implant
    V. Radium removal
   VI. Postradium removal
  VII. Reason to contact physician
VIII. Follow-up

Learner Objectives

    I. The patient describes the hospital routine and states the reasons for hospital policies about radium implant therapy.
      A. A private room and temporary isolation are necessary to decrease radiation exposure to others.
      B. Visitors are generally restricted except for a short time (10 minutes) outside the patient's doorway.
      C. A laundry hamper is kept in the patient's room for collection of possibly radiated linen.
      D. A lead container remains in the room until the radium is removed.
      E. Nursing personnel fulfill the patient's needs quickly and efficiently to keep radiation exposure to a minimum.
   II. The patient describes, in general terms, routine preoperative procedure.
      A. Chest x-ray, EKG, blood work, and urine specimen are obtained.
      B. A cleansing enema may be given, depending on the type of implant and its intended position.
      C. The patient may take nothing by mouth after midnight.
  III. The patient explains the immediate postoperative procedures and the daily routine while the radium is in place.
      A. Vital signs and the position of the radium are checked routinely by nursing personnel to maintain the position of the radium applicator in the uterine canal.

	Content/ Reinforcement Delivered Date & RN	Learner Objectives Met Date & RN	Not Applicable
B. A Foley catheter is inserted to drain urine, keeping the bladder empty and free from the path of radiation.			
C. A constipating pill and a low-residue diet are given to prevent a bowel movement, which could dislodge the applicator. However, if a bowel movement is inevitable, the patient should not strain.			
D. Elastic stockings and injections of a blood thinner (Heparin) are used to prevent blood clots in legs and to improve circulation to the extremities. Circulation is also improved by exercising on a footboard.			
E. "Log rolling" with the legs together is allowed. The head of the bed may be elevated 30°, but the legs may not be flexed.			
F. Bathing is allowed with the exception of pericare.			
G. Strict bedrest is maintained and an air or water mattress is used to increase patient comfort and prevent bedsores.			
IV. The patient describes directions to be followed should the radium become dislodged.			
A. Do not touch or discard any material that may be dislodged.			
B. Do not sit up or get out of bed.			
C. Notify nursing personnel immediately.			
D. Using tongs, the nurse will place the dislodged material into the lead radium container, then notify the doctor.			
V. The patient describes radiation removal procedure.			
A. Radium is removed in the patient's room by the radiologist.			
B. Medication to decrease discomfort may be given before the removal of the radium.			
C. The nurse or doctor can tell the patient exactly when the radium will be removed since the time is determined by computer.			
VI. The patient states the procedure to be followed after the radium is removed.			
A. The Foley catheter is removed and the patient must void a sufficient amount (more than 100 cc) before discharge.			
B. Vital signs are taken lying and sitting to assess dizziness caused by prolonged bedrest.			
C. Sitting with the legs dangling, ambulation and pericare are done with the assistance of the nurse.			
D. The patient may expect diarrhea and frequent vaginal discharge for 2 to 3 weeks.			
VII. The patient states the reasons to call the physician after discharge:			
A. Fever			
B. Bright red vaginal bleeding			

	Content/ Reinforcement Delivered Date & RN	Learner Objectives Met Date & RN	Not Applicable

C. Symptoms of urinary tract infection such as burning, urgency, frequency, blood in the urine
VIII. The patient describes follow-up care:
    A. Appointment with physician
    B. How to contact the physician
        Physician #: _____
        Emergency room # _____			

Evaluation

If patient or significant others are unable to complete some or all of this teaching plan, document evaluation in progress notes.

	Content/ Reinforcement Delivered Date & RN	Learner Objectives Met Date & RN	Not Applicable

VAGINITIS
 	
Purpose
 	
To provide the patient with knowledge about the different types of vaginal infections.
 	
Content
 	
    I. Description of the female anatomy
   II. Discussion of causative factors
 III. Types of vaginal infections
 IV. Medications
  V. Prevention of further infections
 VI. Follow-up			

Learner Objectives
 	
    I. The patient describes the female anatomy related to vaginitis:
      A. Vagina
      B. Urinary meatus
      C. Rectum
   II. The patient discusses the causative factors:
      A. Primary factors (there are none)
      B. Secondary factors
         1. Poor toilet technique
         2. Poor hygiene
         3. Sexual transmission
         4. Frequent douching
         5. Nylon panties or pantyhose
         6. Excess weight
         7. Pregnancy
         8. Diabetes
         9. Use of antibiotics
       10. Birth control pills
       11. Debilitation
 III. The patient states the name of her infection and its signs and symptoms:
      A. Trichomonas
         1. Watery, yellow-greenish discharge (sometimes frothy with a foul odor)
         2. Itching and burning when urinating
         3. Redness
         4. Pain during intercourse
      B. Hemophilus
         1. Discharge that wets underwear
         2. Foul odor or itching			

	Content/ Reinforcement Delivered Date & RN	Learner Objectives Met Date & RN	Not Applicable

3. Itching and burning on urination
   4. Pain or bleeding with intercourse
 C. Monilia (yeast)
   1. Itching
   2. White, cottage cheese–like discharge
   3. Burning on urination
   4. Musty, yeastlike odor
   5. Dryness in vagina when intercourse is attempted
 D. Nonspecific
   1. Itching
   2. Thin, watery discharge
 E. Chlamydia (no known signs or symptoms other than an infection that does not go away)
IV. The patient meets the objectives of the medication teaching plan for prescribed medication.
 V. The patient states how to prevent further infections:
 A. Good hygiene
 B. Front-to-back toilet technique
 C. Cotton underwear, airing of vagina
 D. No douching, deodorant spray, or tampons
 E. Adequate fluid intake
VI. The patient states special follow-up instructions:
 A. Resumption of vaginal intercourse or oral genital sex
 B. Treatment of partner
 C. The patient states follow-up appointment:
 	
_____
 	
 D. Patient states how to contact physician or nurse.
   Physician _____
   Nurse _____
 E. The patient states the reasons or symptoms for which she should contact the physician:
   1. Persistent vaginitis
   2. Discharge
   3. Itching
   4. Painful intercourse
 F. The patient takes home appropriate medication handout.			

Evaluation If patient or significant others are unable to complete some or all of this teaching plan, document evaluation in progress notes.			

GUIDELINES: VAGINITIS

I. The patient describes the female anatomy related to vaginitis. Vaginitis is an infection specific to the vagina. It can be caused by a fungus, parasite, or bacteria. Depending on the type of infection, the organism can be found in the vagina, rectum, or oral cavity. The organisms may be spread by sexual transmission but can also travel by poor toilet technique (wiping from the rectum to the vagina). It is possible to have more than one vaginal infection at the same time.

II. Causative factors.

III. Description of types of vaginitis and its clinical manifestations.

  A. Trichomonas vaginitis ("tric") is caused by the organism *Trichomonas vaginalis*. This organism is normally found in the vagina. It multiplies under certain conditions, causing an infection. Conditions causing it to grow are poor toilet technique, poor hygiene, and frequent douching. Symptoms are (1) a watery, yellow-greenish discharge, (2) itching and burning when urinating, (3) redness, and (4) pain with intercourse.

  B. Hemophilus vaginitis is named for the organism that causes it. This organism is part of the normal vaginal flora. It multiplies under certain conditions, causing an infection. Most often it is transmitted through sexual activity. However, other causes can be poor hygiene, frequent douching, or poor toilet technique. The symptoms of hemophilus vaginitis include (1) a discharge that wets the underwear, (2) foul odor, (3) itching, (4) itching and burning on urination, and (5) pain or bleeding during intercourse. A man can be infected with the hemophilus organism but rarely has symptoms. However, he can reinfect a woman. Because of this, both partners are treated. It is advisable to abstain from vaginal intercourse and oral genital sex or to have the man wear a condom.

  C. Monilia is a yeast: *Candida albicans*. It is found in the normal vaginal flora. It is not known why it causes infections, but certain conditions predispose a woman to monilia. These conditions are pregnancy, diabetes, the use of birth control pills, and use of antibiotics treating another infection. Also, nylon panties and pantyhose and excessive weight prevent airing of the vagina and may cause a monilia infection. Symptoms of a monilia infection are (1) itching, (2) a white, cottage cheese–like discharge, (3) burning on urination, (4) musty, yeastlike odor, and (5) dryness in vagina when intercourse is attempted.

  D. Nonspecific vaginitis has no known organism that causes the infection. Often there is a thin, watery discharge and itching.

  E. Chlamydia is a bacteria found in a variety of places in the body. It can be found in the eyes, ears, respiratory tract, and, in the female, the cervix, urethra, or Fallopian tubes.

V. Explanation of prevention of further infections and considerations during treatment of vaginitis.

  A. It is important that the entire treatment be completed or recurrence of the infection may occur. If menstruation occurs, continue to use medication as directed, but do not use tampons because they absorb the medication. Use sanitary napkins instead.

  B. Abstain from intercourse or oral genital sex until treatment is completed and discomfort is gone. Use of a condom is mandatory to prevent reinfection.

  C. Use good toilet technique (wipe from front to back).

  D. Keep the vaginal area clean and wear all-cotton underwear.

  E. Sometimes the partner must be treated even if he has no symptoms because he can cause reinfection. The provider will make a decision whether to treat both partners.

  F. Drink plenty of fluids like water or juices (not coffee, tea, or soda).

VI. Follow-up care. One restriction often placed on a patient when being treated for a vaginal infection is *not* to engage in vaginal intercourse or oral genital sex during treatment regimen. If abstinence is not possible, the use of a condom is strongly encouraged because most often the infection is transmitted back and forth through sexual activity. A man can be infected but rarely has symptoms. However, he can reinfect a woman. Because of this, both partners are often treated. Specific instructions will be given by the provider to both partners being treated. Follow-up care is necessary or may be done at a routine annual exam. Names and numbers of the nurse and physician are to be given to the patient with instructions to call if she has persistent vaginal discharge, itching, odor, or painful intercourse once the treatment regime has been completed. Appropriate medication handouts should be given to the patient before leaving the clinical area.

BIBLIOGRAPHY

Benson, R.C. (1980). *Handbook of obstetrics and gynecology* (7th ed.). California: Lange Medical Publication.

Lederle Laboratories. (1977). *Service to life: Vaginitis questions and answers*. New York: Author.

Merrell-National Laboratories. (1973). *A woman explains vaginitis*. Ohio: Author.

Smith Kline Clinical Laboratories. (1981). *Culture for Chlamydia—Test information*. Boston: Author.

Part VIII

The Respiratory System

	Content/ Reinforcement Delivered Date & RN	Learner Objectives Met Date & RN	Not Applicable

ASTHMA

Purpose

To increase the patient and family's knowledge of asthma, its causative factors, clinical manifestations, complications, and treatment.
To ensure greater compliance with maintenance and management of disease.
To prevent progression of disease.

Content

    I. Description of normal lung anatomy and physiology
   II. Description of asthma and its causes
  III. Physiology of asthma
  IV. Clinical manifestations
   V. Medications
  VI. Bronchial hygiene measures
 VII. Environmental control
VIII. Handout
  IX. Psychological aspects

Learner Objectives

    I. The patient describes the normal anatomy and physiology of the lungs.
       A. The lungs are two saclike organs located in the chest cavity.
       B. The main function of the lungs is to supply oxygen to the blood and to remove carbon dioxide from the blood.
       C. Unobstructed air passages are required for the lungs to perform this function successfully.
       D. Air enters through the mouth and nose and travels into the lungs by airways known as *bronchi*. These bronchi branch, or divide, into smaller airways as a tree divides into small branches. The smallest airways are very small and are found in groups known as *alveoli*.
       E. The walls of the alveoli contain small blood vessels known as *capillaries*.
       F. Oxygen passes from the alveoli to the capillaries and is then carried throughout the body by the blood. Carbon dioxide is passed from the capillaries to the alveoli in the lungs and then the carbon dioxide is exhaled.
   II. The patient describes asthma and its causes.
       A. Asthma is a disease characterized by recurrent episodes of wheezing, shortness of breath, and coughing.

	Content/ Reinforcement Delivered Date & RN	Learner Objectives Met Date & RN	Not Applicable

B. Precipitants of asthmatic attacks are known irritants such as
  1. Allergens
  2. Infection
  3. Cold air
  4. Cigarette smoke
III. The patient lists physiologic changes of asthma.
  A. Spasm of the muscles of the bronchial tubes leads to narrowing of the tubes.
  B. Lining cells of the bronchial tubes swell and produce increased amounts of mucus.
IV. The patient states clinical manifestations of asthma:
  A. Wheezing, caused by air flowing through narrowed airways
  B. Shortness of breath, due to the increased work one must do to breathe through narrowed airways
  C. Cough, due to the irritation of the airways because of swelling and mucous secretions
  D. Sputum production, due to increased mucous production
V. The patient meets the objectives of the medication teaching plan for each medication prescribed.
VI. The patient describes and demonstrates appropriate bronchial hygiene measures:
  A. Breathing exercises
    1. Purpose of breathing exercises
      a) To minimize asthma attacks
      b) To increase the patient's confidence and control during an attack
      c) To reduce the sensation of dyspnea by reducing the amount of energy expended by increasing breathing efficiency
    2. Example of a breathing exercise
      a) Sit in a chair with arms.
      b) Place one hand over the stomach (epigastric area below the breastbone).
      c) Push manually in and up on stomach during expiration (causes upward movement of diaphragm).
      d) Concentrate on a slow, deep expiration.
      e) Relax manual pressure on the stomach during inspiration.
      f) A deeper inspiration will usually follow.
    3. Caution to be exhibited during an asthma attack
      a) Airway resistance is increased during an asthma attack.
      b) Discourage forced expiration, as this will only increase airway resistance.			

	Content/ Reinforcement Delivered Date & RN	Learner Objectives Met Date & RN	Not Applicable

    c) Emphasis should be on slowing the *rate* of expiration and improving the depth.

    d) This pattern will help keep the airway open longer, thereby increasing ventilation and aeration.

B. Postural drainage and percussion

  1. This technique uses gravity (posturing) and chest physical therapy (cupping, clapping, deep breathing, assisted coughing, and vibration) to relieve airway obstruction caused by excessive amounts of secretions.

  2. Patient meets objectives of postural drainage teaching plan.

C. Cool mist humidifier

  1. Adds cool humidity to air

  2. Prevents dehydration of airways and thus helps prevent the subsequent increased susceptibility to infection

  3. May be purchased at drug or department stores

VII. The patient describes potential and existing environmental factors that should be avoided.

A. Avoid dust collectors such as chenille bedspreads, heavy curtains, thick and shaggy rugs, books, stuffed animals, or knick-knacks.

B. Avoid dark, damp areas that potentiate mold growth such as damp cellars or bathrooms.

C. Avoid irritating fumes such as smoke, deodorants, and some cooking or cleaning fumes.

D. Do not sweep with a broom, as this stimulates dust. Always damp mop by using a damp rag strapped around the broom to pick up dust.

E. Do not dust with a feather duster or dry cloth. Always spray with a fine mist or water over the surface and damp dust.

F. Always air out the house after cleaning.

G. Wear a mask while cleaning house.

VIII. Patient takes home handout on environmental control.

IX. The patient describes the psychological implications of his illness:

A. The relationship between asthma and the psyche

  1. It is popular belief that asthma is psychosomatic in origin.

  2. Emotionally stressful situations may precipitate episodes, but there is little evidence that emotional distress can be the sole etiological factor.

  3. As in any chronic disease, emotional problems can aggravate the disease and prolong its symptoms.

	Content/ Reinforcement Delivered Date & RN	Learner Objectives Met Date & RN	Not Applicable

4. Prolonged bouts of asthma can cause additional emotional stress.
B. Appropriate interventions
   1. The patient should try to avoid stressful situations.
   2. The patient identifies coping mechanisms when stress is unavoidable.
 	
Evaluation
 	
If patient or significant others are unable to complete some or all of this teaching plan, document evaluation in progress notes.			

	Content/ Reinforcement Delivered	Learner Objectives Met	Not Applicable
	Date & RN	Date & RN	

CHRONIC OBSTRUCTIVE PULMONARY DISEASE (COPD)

Purpose

To increase patient and family's knowledge of COPD, its causative factors, clinical manifestations, complications, and treatment.
To ensure greater compliance with maintenance and management of disease.

Content

   I. Description of normal lung anatomy and physiology
  II. Description of COPD: chronic bronchitis and emphysema
 III. Causes of chronic bronchitis and emphysema
 IV. Physiologic changes of chronic bronchitis and emphysema
  V. Clinical manifestations of chronic bronchitis and emphysema
 VI. Medication
VII. Bronchial hygiene measures
VIII. Common home equipment
 IX. Health care providers involved with patient care
  X. Diagram of parts of lung and pursed lip breathing
 XI. Reasons to call physician
XII. Follow-up

Learner Objectives

  I. The patient describes the normal anatomy and physiology of the lungs.
    A. The lungs are two saclike organs located in the chest cavity.
    B. The main function of the lungs is to supply oxygen to the blood and to remove carbon dioxide from the blood.
    C. It is important to keep the air passages clear so proper exchange of gases can take place.
    D. Air enters the body through the nose and mouth and travels down the windpipe (trachea) into the smaller airways (bronchi and bronchioles). At the end of the small airways are tiny clusters called *alveoli* (air sacs).
    E. Around each air sac are small blood vessels called *capillaries*.
    F. The passage of gases takes place between the air sacs and the capillaries. With an increase in secretions, breathing becomes more difficult because the secretions interfere with the flow of air.

	Content/ Reinforcement Delivered Date & RN	Learner Objectives Met Date & RN	Not Applicable

II. The patient describes COPD, chronic bronchitis, and emphysema. (See Figures 5 and 6.)
   A. COPD is the severe blockage of air flow during expiration due to the narrowing of the airways. Several diseases may cause COPD, such as chronic bronchitis and emphysema.
   B. Chronic bronchitis is an increase in the amount of sputum in the bronchial tree. The patient has a productive cough for 3 months per year for at least 2 years.
   C. Emphysema is the enlargement of the alveoli. Air becomes trapped in them, which makes breathing more difficult.
III. The patient states two causes of chronic bronchitis and emphysema:
   A. Infection
   B. Chronic irritation due to cigarette smoking, air pollution, dusts, allergies
IV. The patient states physiologic changes of chronic bronchitis and emphysema.
   A. With chronic bronchitis the lining of the airways becomes swollen and excessive mucus is produced, making it more difficult for air to get in and out of the lungs.
   B. With emphysema the large air spaces weaken the walls of the airways, thus making it more difficult to exhale.
V. The patient describes clinical manifestations of chronic bronchitis and emphysema.
   A. The patient names four manifestations of chronic bronchitis:
     1. Increase in cough and sputum production
     2. Frequent respiratory infections followed by a cough
     3. Increase in thickness of the sputum
     4. Increase in shortness of breath
   B. The patient describes two manifestations of emphysema:
     1. Difficult expiration
     2. Increase in shortness of breath on exertion
VI. The patient meets the objectives of the medication teaching plan for each medication.
VII. The patient describes and demonstrates bronchial hygiene measures (see Figure 7).
   A. The patient states the purpose of breathing exercises.
     1. Patients with COPD breathe rapidly and inefficiently, forcing wasted air into over-inflated lungs.
     2. The patient describes breathing exercises (see Figure 7).
       a) Count to 3 on inhalation.
       b) Relax.		

	Content/ Reinforcement Delivered	Learner Objectives Met	Not Applicable
	Date & RN	Date & RN	

  c) Expand abdomen.
  d) Purse lips and begin to exhale.
  e) Count to 6 or 7.
  f) Contract abdominal muscles during exhalation.
  g) If having difficulty, lean forward (i.e., tying shoes or picking up an object). This aids in exhalation.
B. The patient states the purpose, describes and demonstrates the controlled coughing technique.
  1. With COPD there is an increase in sputum; therefore, it is important to learn the most effective way to cough.
  2. The patient demonstrates six steps for controlled coughing.
    a) Take a slow deep breath.
    b) Hold deep breath for 2 seconds.
    c) Cough twice with mouth slightly opened. The first cough loosens the secretions, the second moves it forward.
    d) Pause.
    e) Inhale by sniffing gently.
    f) Rest.
  3. Helpful hints. The patient makes a hollow sound with correct coughing. Have the patient drink a glass of water before coughing. This will loosen secretions.
C. The patient names five times when postural drainage and percussion should be done:
  1. An increase in secretions
  2. Thick and sticky secretions
  3. Difficulty in coughing up secretions
  4. Poor, ineffective cough
  5. Weakness of breathing muscles
D. If appropriate, the patient meets the objectives of the postural drainage teaching plan.
E. The patient states adequate hydration can be provided by
  1. Drinking eight glasses of fluid a day. If on fluid restriction, check with the physician.
  2. Steam inhalations two to five times a day to keep secretions loose and liquid.
F. The patient states the importance of increasing exercise and activity, i.e., walking short distances and resting for 15-minute intervals, then continuing with exercise.
VIII. The patient discusses common home equipment:
A. IPPB machine (Intermittent Positive Pressure Breathing). This machine blows air into the lungs and opens

	Content/ Reinforcement Delivered Date & RN	Learner Objectives Met Date & RN	Not Applicable

the air sacs so secretions will loosen and can be coughed up.

B. Nebulizer mask. This produces a mist to loosen secretions in the lungs when the patient breathes.

C. Oxygen
  1. Types
    a) Oxygen cylinder. Tank with a gauge that identifies when the oxygen level is low. A smaller cylinder can be carried by a shoulder strap.
    b) Oxygen concentration. The machine takes in room air and generates oxygen.
    c) Liquid oxygen. The patient is able to transfer liquid oxygen from a large cylinder to smaller cylinder and carry it with a portable shoulder strap.
  2. Things to remember about oxygen at home
    a) Do not smoke when using oxygen.
    b) Use only the amount of oxygen ordered by the physician.
    c) Do not move the cylinder.
    d) Do not try to repair the equipment.
    e) Call the oxygen company if the gauge indicates 500 pounds of oyxgen left.

IX. The patient states how to contact the following professionals involved in care:

A. Primary nurse
  Name: _____
  Phone #: _____

B. Physician
  Name: _____
  Phone #: _____

C. Respiratory therapist
  Name: _____
  Phone #: _____

D. Home oxygen company
  Name: _____
  Phone #: _____

X. The patient explains the diagram attached to the teaching plan.

XI. The patient states reasons to contact the physician:
A. Change in sputum
B. Fever
C. Increased congestion
D. Abnormal change in breathing

	Content/ Reinforcement Delivered Date & RN	Learner Objectives Met Date & RN	Not Applicable

XII. The patient states follow-up appointment:
    Month: _____
    Date: _____
    Time: _____
    Where: _____
 	
Evaluation
 	
If patient or significant others are unable to complete some or all of this teaching plan, document evaluation in progress notes.			

Figure 5 Normal and Obstructed Bronchiole

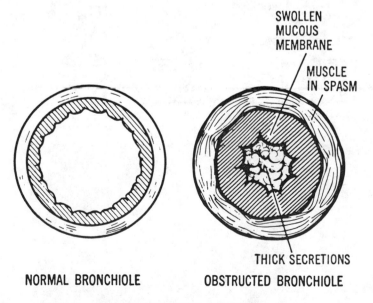

SWOLLEN MUCOUS MEMBRANE

MUSCLE IN SPASM

THICK SECRETIONS

NORMAL BRONCHIOLE   OBSTRUCTED BRONCHIOLE

ENLARGED CROSS SECTION

Figure 6 Normal and Broken-Down Alveoli

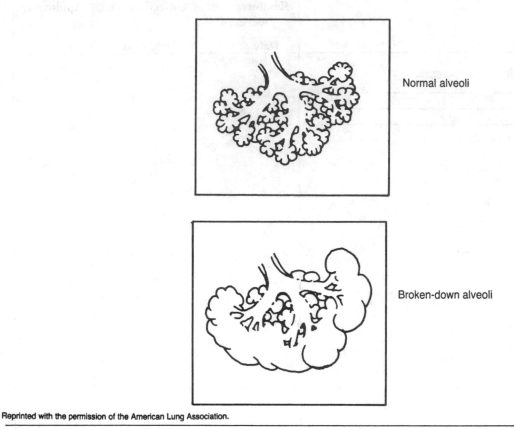

Normal alveoli

Broken-down alveoli

Figure 7 Bronchial Hygiene Measure

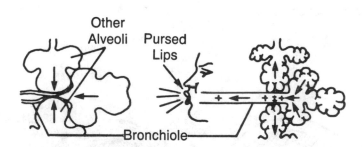

	Content/ Reinforcement Delivered Date & RN	Learner Objectives Met Date & RN	Not Applicable

PEDIATRIC PATIENT WITH PNEUMONIA

Purpose

To provide the child and family with a knowledge of pneumonia, its implications, and treatment.

Content

    I. Definition of pneumonia
    II. Characteristics of pneumonia
    III. Signs and symptoms of pneumonia
    IV. Medications used to treat pneumonia
    V. Diagnostic tests
    VI. Description of treatments
    VII. Instruction for discharge
    VIII. Reasons to contact physician

Learner Objectives

    I. Patient and parent define pneumonia.
       A. Pneumonia is an infection that enters the lungs through the respiratory passages, causing them to fill with fluid and become congested.
    II. The family describes the characteristics of pneumonia.
       A. Pneumonia may occur alone or in addition to other medical problems.
       B. Medical problems that cause a child to be more susceptible to pneumonia are cleft palate, muscular dystrophy, and immune deficiency.
       C. Pneumonia can be classified according to causative agent (bacterial or viral) and according to the area of the lung involved (lobar, bronchial, etc.).
       D. The highest incidence of pneumonia is found in children under 5 years of age.
       E. Most bacterial and viral pneumonias occur during winter and spring.
       F. Treatment of pneumonia is aimed at killing the organism with antibiotics if bacterial and clearing the lungs of congestion, which will assist the child in breathing more easily.
    III. The patient and parents identify the signs and symptoms of pneumonia.
       A. Elevated temperature and elevated heart rate are common.
       B. Elevated respiratory rate is often accompanied by retractions or a pulling in of the abdominal muscles when trying to breathe.

	Content/ Reinforcement Delivered	Learner Objectives Met	Not Applicable
	Date & RN	Date & RN	
C. Dry hacking cough progresses to a looser cough with an increase in sputum.			
D. A change in color may occur. Child may become dusky or bluish around the mouth, nailbeds, or mucous membranes. Patient may also be slightly grayish, depending on the need for oxygen.			
E. The child may experience upper respiratory symptoms, stuffy nose, irritability, etc. These often precede the onset of pneumonia.			
F. Other frequent symptoms include a decrease in appetite, nausea, vomiting, and diarrhea. The child may also be extremely lethargic and irritable.			
IV. If medications are being used to treat the child in the hospital, parents identify and describe these medications: A. Name: _____ B. Route: _____ C. Action: _____			

V. The child and parents state the diagnostic tests and describe how they are used to monitor the child's condition:
 A. Frequent blood sampling
   1. To determine if pneumonia is viral or bacterial
   2. To determine what organism is present and what antibiotics it is sensitive to
   3. To follow progress of the infection and its response to the chosen medication
 B. Chest x-rays
   1. To show the location of the pneumonia
   2. To determine if improvement or worsening of pneumonia is occurring
 C. Frequent vital signs and assessment of breath sounds
   1. To monitor changes in temperature, heart rate, or respiratory rate
   2. To determine the location and thickness of secretions in the lungs, which allows the doctor to concentrate treatment on these areas			

VI. Patient and parents explain the reasons for specific treatments being used. A. Intravenous fluids may be needed to maintain adequate hydration and administer antibiotics. B. A mist tent is used to moisten the respiratory tract. C. Oxygen aids in supplying additional oxygen to the blood when the diseased part of the lung is unable to do so, thus enabling the child to breathe more easily. D. Postural drainage helps loosen secretions from lung walls to reexpand collapsed areas of the lung and relieve congestion.			

	Content/ Reinforcement Delivered Date & RN	Learner Objectives Met Date & RN	Not Applicable
E. Suction is used when the child is unable to cough up secretions. If left in the lungs, they would cause more infection.			
VII. Parents complete teaching plan and state special instructions for discharge.			
A. Complete the medication teaching plan for all major discharge medications			
B. Describe treatments to be done at home:			
1. Postural drainage (completes teaching plan)			
2. Mist tent or vaporizer			
VIII. Parents state reasons and procedure for contacting physician:			
A. Recurring signs and symptoms of pneumonia			
1. Elevation of temperature, heart rate, or respiratory rate, which may be accompanied by increased difficulty in breathing. Note any changes in skin color.			
2. Dry hacking cough with increased sputum production.			
3. Stuffy nose, irritability, and decrease in appetite. May also be followed by nausea, vomiting, and diarrhea.			
B. Difficulties administering medications or treatments			
C. Date, time, and place of the follow-up visit with the doctor or clinic, with all the necessary appointment cards and phone numbers: Date: ____ Time: ____ Physician #: ____ Emergency room #: ____			

Evaluation

If patient or significant others are unable to complete some or all of this teaching plan, document evaluation in progress notes.

	Content/ Reinforcement Delivered Date & RN	Learner Objectives Met Date & RN	Not Applicable

POSTURAL DRAINAGE
 	
Purpose
 	
To teach the patients and their families the purpose and proper method of postural drainage.
 	
Content
 	
    I. Definition of postural drainage (PD)
   II. Simple anatomy and physiology of lungs
  III. Purpose and method of cupping and vibration
  IV. Purpose and method of different positions used for postural drainage
   V. Time requirements for postural drainage
  VI. Importance of coughing
 VII. Signs and symptoms of tiring and distress
VIII. Evaluation and follow-up		

Learner Objectives
 	
    I. Patient and significant other correctly define postural drainage.
       A. Specific body positions and percussion are used so that the force of gravity can assist in reexpanding collapsed areas of the lung.
       B. Postural drainage mobilizes and removes bronchial secretions from the lungs of patients who are having difficulty coughing up secretions on their own.
   II. Patient and significant other describe in simple terms the anatomy of the lungs.
      A. The lungs are two balloonlike organs located within the chest.
         1. The right lung is composed of three lobes or sections: right upper lobe (RUL), right middle lobe (RML), and right lower lobe (RLL).
         2. The left lung is made up of only two lobes: left upper lobe (LUL) and the left lower lobe (LLL).
  III. After instruction by the nurse, the patient and significant other demonstrate that the proper method for cupping or percussion is a tapping of the chest in a firm and rapid manner over the lobe being treated.
      A. Cupping is done holding the hand in a cupped manner with all the fingertips and thumbs together.
      B. In a small infant, cupping is done by holding two or three fingertips together and lightly tapping the chest.		

	Content/ Reinforcement Delivered	Learner Objectives Met	Not Applicable
	Date & RN	**Date & RN**	

    C. This percussion dislodges plugs and mucus from the lungs. It stimulates the patient to cough, which helps bring up the secretions.

    D. Vibration is a maneuver done after clapping that stimulates the flow of secretions.

    E. To vibrate, the hand must be kept flat and pressed firmly against the proper segment of the patient's chest wall.

    F. One vibration directed from the flattened hand to the chest wall should be applied while the patient exhales slowly. This may be repeated as the patient tolerates.

IV. Patient and significant other correctly define the purpose and demonstrate the proper method of postural drainage for all lobes. (See Figure 8.)

    A. Upper lobes

        1. Place patient in upright position by elevating head of bed approximately 30° to 45° or if the patient is a small child, place the child in your lap.

        2. The front portions of both lobes are percussed at the same time in an alternating rhythmic manner over the upper part of the chest directly below the clavicle.

        3. For the rear segments of the upper lobes, place the patient on stomach and percuss the back in the same way as the front segments.

    B. Right middle lobe

        1. Place the patient flat in bed or if a child, on your lap lying on the child's left side.

        2. Percussing is performed over the front, back, and side portion of the lobe. This is done at about the same level as the nipple line and directly under the armpit.

    C. Right lower lobe (RLL) and left lower lobe (LLL)

        1. For the RLL, place the patient on the left side with head lower than feet at a 45° angle either on your lap or in bed with two pillows under the hips. For the LLL, use same position with the patient lying on the right side.

        2. Percuss over the front, back, and side portion of the lobe at the level of the lower ribs.

V. Patient and significant other state the best time to perform postural drainage and the proper amount of time to be spent on each lobe.

    A. Postural drainage should not be done before or after meals.

        1. Half hour rest should be allowed before patient's scheduled mealtime.

	Content/ Reinforcement Delivered Date & RN	Learner Objectives Met Date & RN	Not Applicable

2. To avoid vomiting, wait at least 1 hour after meal-time.
B. The average time for percussion of each lobe is at least 1 minute.
  1. The length of time depends on the level of tolerance of each patient.
  2. The time spent on postural drainage also depends on severity of the patient's condition.
 	
VI. Patient and significant other explain the importance of coughing during and after postural drainage.
  A. Coughing is an essential part of clearing the airways.
  B. It helps bring up secretions that have been loosened and removed from the walls of the lungs while receiving postural drainage.
  C. Patient should take one to two deep breaths and then cough as exhaling.
  D. Coughing should be done during postural drainage and after each lobe has had proper postural drainage.
 	
VII. Patient and significant other identify the signs and symptoms of tiring and distress. It should be noted whether
  A. The patient has labored respirations and increased difficulty breathing.
  B. The patient's color is poor: either a bluish color to the skin or pallor.
  C. The patient sounds increasingly congested.
 	
VIII. Patient and significant other identify how progress will be evaluated.
  A. If visiting nurses visit the home, they can evaluate and assist with postural drainage. They can also listen to breath sounds and evaluate patient's progress.
  B. If follow-up appointment is arranged, the patient states
    1. Date: _____
    2. Time: _____
      a) On visit to the physician, breath sounds are assessed again as well as the patient's respiratory rate. Chest x-rays may also be taken to evaluate respiratory status further.
      b) If patient needs to be seen before the appointment or has questions, the patient has the necessary phone numbers to reach physician, nurse or clinic
      Physician: _____
      Nurse: _____
      Clinic: _____		

	Content/ Reinforcement Delivered Date & RN	Learner Objectives Met Date & RN	Not Applicable
Evaluation If patient or significant others are unable to complete some or all of this teaching plan, document evaluation in progress notes.			

Figure 8 Postural Drainage Positions

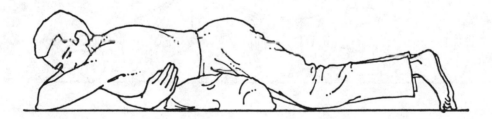

POSITION 1
Lying face downward with pillow under lower abdomen. Drains portion of lower lobe. (Clap over lower ribs.)*

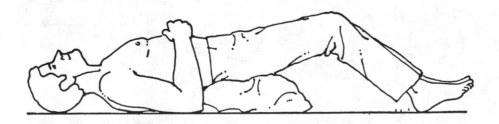

POSITION 2
Lying on back with pillow under hips. Drains anterior (front) portion of chest. (Clap over lower ribs.)*

Figure 8 continued

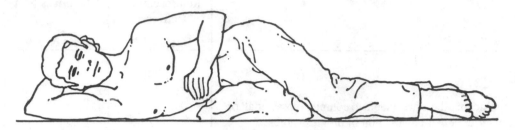

POSITION
3
Lying on right side, pillow under lower abdomen. Drains left lower lobe. (Clap over lower ribs.)*

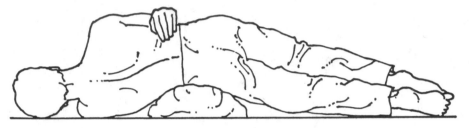

POSITION
4
Lying on left side, pillow under lower abdomen. Drains right lower lobe. (Clap over lower ribs.)*

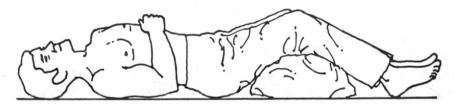

POSITION
5
Lying on back, slightly turned to one side, pillow under knees. Drains anterior basal (front lower) segment of lower lobe. (Clap over lower ribs.)*

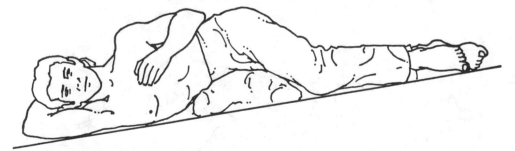

POSITION
6
Lying on right side, feet higher than head, pillow between hip bone and bottom ribs. Drains lingular (equivalent to left middle lobe) segment. (Clap over left nipple area.)*

*If clapping is ordered by your physician.

Source: Reprinted from *Postural Drainage Positions*, Breon Laboratories Inc., New York, NY.

	Content/ Reinforcement Delivered Date & RN	Learner Objectives Met Date & RN	Not Applicable

THORACOTOMY

Purpose

To help the patient understand the preoperative and postoperative events of the thoractomy procedure.
To reduce anxiety and enhance patient cooperation during the preoperative and postoperative phases.

Content

I. Reason for thoractomy
II. Description of the procedure
III. Explanation of preoperative events
IV. Explanation of postoperative events
V. Reasons to stop smoking
VI. Normal events during recovery
VII. Reasons to contact physician
VIII. How to contact physician
IX. Follow-up

Learner Objectives

I. The patient describes the reasons for a thoractomy.
II. The patient describes a thoractomy.

III. The patient describes preoperative events.
   A. Smoking is discouraged because smoking increases bronchial irritation, thereby increasing secretions.
   B. Chest x-ray, ECG, blood work, urine specimens, and pulmonary function tests are done to establish a pre-operative baseline.
   C. Anterior and posterior chest scrubs are done with an antibacterial soap to prepare the skin for surgery.
   D. The chest physiotherapist visits and demonstrates proper breathing exercises and use of the incentive spirometer for postoperative use.
   E. Preoperative medication is given to reduce anxiety. Antibiotics are given at midnight and at 6 AM the day of surgery to prevent infection postoperatively.
   F. Transportation to the operating room is provided via stretcher; jewelry or dentures are removed and a hospital gown put on.

	Content/ Reinforcement Delivered Date & RN	Learner Objectives Met Date & RN	Not Applicable
IV. The patient describes postoperative events. 　A. The patient remains in the recovery room until awake and the tube that assists with breathing is taken out of the throat. 　B. The incision is covered with a heavy dressing. 　C. Chest tubes are inserted to permit the drainage of air and fluid from the area surrounding the lung (the pleural space). The tubes make a soft, bubbling noise. 　D. Coughing, deep breathing, and incentive spirometer exercises are encouraged to help move secretions out of the lungs and assist in reexpanding the lungs. 　E. There is pain from the incision and from the presence of the chest tubes. There may be pain, numbness, or heaviness in the operative region. Medication is provided to help decrease pain. 　F. Arm exercises are encouraged several times a day to prevent arm and shoulder stiffness. V. The patient states reasons to stop smoking permanently: 　A. To decrease bronchial secretions 　B. To reduce further lung disease VI. The patient states that weakness and fatigue are common 3 to 4 weeks postoperatively. Pain gradually decreases, but an analgesic and warm soaks to the operative area may help. VII. The patient states reasons for contacting the doctor: 　A. Temperature above 99°F. 　B. Drainage from the incision 　C. Shortness of breath 　D. Bloody sputum VIII. The patient states how to contact the doctor: 　A. Physician #: _____ 　B. Emergency room #: _____ IX. The patient states the date and time of follow-up appointment: 　A. Date: _____ 　B. Time: _____ **Evaluation** If patient or significant others are unable to complete some or all of this teaching plan, document evaluation in progress notes.			

	Content/ Reinforcement Delivered Date & RN	Learner Objectives Met Date & RN	Not Applicable

HOME CARE FOR TRACHEOTOMY: ADULT

(To be used with Tracheal Suctioning plan)

Purpose

To teach the patient and family to care for the tracheotomy at home.

Content

   I. Anatomy and physiology of the respiratory system
  II. Parts of a tracheotomy tube
 III. Methods of cleaning a tracheotomy tube
 IV. Use of humidification
  V. Communication
 VI. Review of tracheotomy booklet
VII. Extra tube
VIII. How and when to contact the physician
 IX. Follow-up

Learner Objectives

  I. The patient describes the anatomy of the respiratory system.
     A. Review a diagram with the patient so that the patient can identify
        1. Tongue
        2. Epiglottis
        3. Trachea (passage to lungs)
        4. Vocal chords
        5. Esophagus (passage to stomach)
     B. The patient points out on a picture where the tube is in relation to the airway.
 II. The patient describes the parts of a tracheotomy tube.
     A. Using an extra tube, the patient identifies each part and its function:
        1. Outer tube. The outer tube maintains the airway opening and should be removed only with special permission of physician.
        2. Inner tube. The inner tube may be removed daily and whenever necessary for cleaning. It maintains a clear airway.
        3. Obturator. The obturator is used only for insertion of tube and should be kept with the tube as a complete set.
        4. Lock. Patient demonstrates how the inner and outer tube lock together so that the inner tube remains in place.

	Content/ Reinforcement Delivered Date & RN	Learner Objectives Met Date & RN	Not Applicable

III. The patient describes the method of cleaning a tracheotomy tube.
 	
    A. The patient identifies equipment needed:
      1. Bowl
      2. Small brush
      3. Cotton tape
      4. Gauze sponges (without filler)
      5. Tracheotomy dressing
      6. Water and hydrogen peroxide
 	
    B. The patient demonstrates step-by-step cleaning of the tube by clean technique.
      1. Washes hands.
      2. Positions self with a mirror in a comfortable position.
      3. Suctions if necessary.
      4. Removes inner tube.
      5. Scrubs inner tube with hydrogen peroxide and brush.
      6. Rinses inner tube with water.
      7. Examines both ends of inner tube for remaining secretions.
      8. Replaces inner tube.
      9. Locks inner tube in place.
      10. Washes hands.
 	
    C. The patient demonstrates how to change the tracheotomy dressing.
      1. Removes old dressing.
      2. Cleans around the stoma with gauze and warm water.
      3. Applies a small amount of Vaseline or Bacitracin on the skin around the tube.
      4. Applies a new dressing.
 	
    D. The patient demonstrates how to change tracheotomy.
      1. Prepares new cotton ties.
      2. Cuts old ties while holding on to the tube.
      3. Removes old ties while holding the tube in place.
      4. Strings new ties in place.
      5. Ties new ties in a knot.
      6. Changes ties whenever necessary.
 	
    E. The patient states variations in cleaning for Portex tube (cuffed tube without an inner tube).
      1. The patient will not remove the tube and scrub it.
      2. The patient demonstrates how to inflate and deflate the cuff.
      3. The patient identifies in instruction booklet which steps are applicable.			

	Content/ Reinforcement Delivered Date & RN	Learner Objectives Met Date & RN	Not Applicable

IV. The patient describes the use of humidification.
  A. The patient states that extra humidification is necessary because air is not being humidified naturally by the nose and mouth.
  B. The patient states what type of extra humidification will be obtained (e.g., cool air, room vaporizer, ultrasonic nebulizer).
V. The patient demonstrates proper communication.
  A. When appropriate, the patient will hold a finger over the tracheotomy when exhaling to speak.
  B. When appropriate, patient will use a pen and paper.
VI. The patient will keep the instruction booklet handy to use as reference at home ("Caring for your Tracheotomy at Home" may be obtained from the ear, nose, and throat clinic).
VII. The patient describes how to use an extra tracheotomy tube.
  A. The patient is given a duplicate tracheotomy tube to take home.
  B. The patient states that if respiratory difficulty is unrelieved by routine measures (e.g., suctioning, cleaning tube), the patient should take the extra tube to the *nearest* emergency room.
VIII. The patient states how and when to contact the physician.
  A. The patient should contact the physician when
    1. Having difficulty breathing
    2. Bleeding from or around the tracheotomy
    3. The quality of secretions changes
    4. Unable to replace the inner tube
    5. Skin around the tube becomes swollen, red, or painful
  B. The patient identifies how to call the hospital and contact primary physician.
IX. The patient states the reason for follow-up appointment and its date.
  A. The patient understands the need to change the tube every month.
  B. The patient states the next appointment: _____			

Evaluation If patient or significant others are unable to complete some or all of this teaching plan, document evaluation in progress notes.			

GUIDELINES: TRACHEOTOMY HOME CARE

I. The patient describes the anatomy of the respiratory system.
   Review a diagram with the patient, especially the relationship of the tracheotomy tube to the trachea and the mechanism of speaking by occluding the tracheotomy tube on expiration.

II. The patient describes the parts of a tracheotomy tube.
   Review the parts of the tracheotomy tube with patient:
   1. Outer tube, which should be removed only with special permission of the physician
   2. Inner tube, which is removed and cleaned to maintain clear airway
   3. Obturator, which is used initially to insert the tube and should be kept with the complete set

III. The patient describes the method of cleaning a tracheotomy tube.
   Cleaning the tracheotomy tube
   1. Equipment
      Bowl
      Small brush
      Cotton tape
      Gauze sponges (without filler)
      Tracheotomy dressing
      Water or hydrogen peroxide
   2. Demonstrate method of removing, cleaning, and replacing inner tube to patient and family. Provide the patient with a small mirror at the bedside or use the bathroom mirror. Wash hands, then suction if necessary. Turn the notch on the inner tube to the correct slot and remove the inner tube following the curvature. Clean the inner tube in hydrogen peroxide or water with a brush. Examine the inside of the tube from both ends to be sure that no secretions remain. Rinse the inner tube and shake off excess water. Replace the inner tube following the curvature to allow for ease of insertion. Turn the notch to lock. Encourage the patient to assist with each part of the procedure gradually until able to complete the entire process. Explain the use of clean instead of sterile technique and stress handwashing before and after the procedure.
   3. Remove tracheotomy dressing. Clean around the stoma with a gauze sponge and warm water. Dry thoroughly. Apply Vaseline or Bacitracin ointment if the skin is reddened from secretions. Replace tracheotomy tape (1-inch tape is easiest). The tracheotomy tape need be replaced only when necessary. Replace tracheotomy dressing, being sure it is completely under the tracheotomy tube.

Provide the patient with enough equipment to begin home care and discuss where future equipment can be obtained:
      Tracheotomy care set or small brush
      Hydrogen peroxide
      Tracheotomy dressings (ask local pharmacy to order)
      Tracheotomy tape (cloth sewing tape)
      Gauze sponges without filler (local pharmacy)
   4. The schedule for cleaning the tracheotomy should depend on amount of secretions. The tracheotomy dressing need not be changed each time. The entire tracheotomy tube should be changed monthly. This is usually done at an outpatient appointment and should be done by the patient at home only with permission of the doctor and after successfully performing the procedure under supervision.

IV. The patient describes the use of humidification. Discuss the importance of humidification since air is breathed directly into the lungs rather than being humidified naturally by breathing through the nose. Plan with the patient the type of humidifier to be used and where it should be placed (e.g., cool air room vaporizer at bedside at night).

V. The patient demonstrates proper communication. Review the method of speaking with the patient if appropriate. The patient should inhale, cover the tracheotomy opening with a finger, and speak on expiration.

VII. The patient describes how to use an extra tracheotomy tube.
   Review tips to remember using "Caring for Your Tracheotomy at Home" booklet. Provide a duplicate tracheotomy tube for the patient to take home. If the patient experiences respiratory difficulty that cannot be relieved, the patient should take this duplicate tube to a local emergency room.

VIII. The patient states how and when to contact the physician. The patient should contact the physician
   1. If bleeding or there is a change in the quality of secretions
   2. If unable to replace the inner tube
   3. If breathing is difficult (go to a local emergency room)
   4. If the skin opening becomes painful, redness increases, or the opening changes in size

IX. The physician's telephone number and the means to contact the resident on call at night or weekends (if appropriate) should be given to the patient. The patient should have a scheduled follow-up appointment with the physician.

Variations for the Portex tube

1. Delete steps for cleaning the inner tube (steps B.4. and 5.)
2. Demonstrate the method of inflating and deflating the cuff.
3. Humidification is especially important, as the Portex tube has no inner tube. It may be necessary to arrange for an ultrasonic nebulizer to be used via tracheotomy mask at home. Use the respiratory therapy department as a resource.
4. The Portex tube should be changed every month in the hospital.
5. In using the "Caring for Your Tracheotomy at Home" booklet, point out to the patient that not all the procedures listed are applicable.

	Content/ Reinforcement Delivered	Learner Objectives Met	Not Applicable
	Date & RN	Date & RN	

TRACHEAL SUCTIONING HOME CARE—CLEAN TECHNIQUE

(To be used with ''Home Care for Tracheotomy'')

Purpose

To remove accumulated tracheal secretions and maintain a patent airway.

Content

   I. Anatomy and physiology of the airway and lungs
  II. Equipment
 III. Use of equipment
 IV. Suctioning procedure
  V. Care of the equipment
 VI. When suctioning is necessary
VII. Methods to relieve difficult breathing

Learner Objectives

   I. The patient describes the anatomy and physiology of the airway.
     A. Using a diagram, the patient identifies important components of the airway.
     B. The patient explains that stimulation of the tracheal wall will produce a cough.
     C. The patient explains how secretions can be coughed orally around the tube on occasion.
  II. Patient identifies the equipment needed:
     A. Suction machine
     B. Suction catheters and a cover
     C. Connecting tubing
     D. Container of water
 III. The patient describes the correct use of the equipment. Turn on the machine, check its function (suctioning water), and demonstrate the suction cut-off control.
 IV. The patient describes or demonstrates the suctioning procedure to the nurse:
     A. Coughing before suctioning to improve suctioning.
     B. Insertion of the catheter (only to the length of the tracheotomy tube). The patient may use a mirror for guiding the insertion.
     C. Covering the suction cut-off with the thumb to start suctioning.
     D. Rotation of the catheter while withdrawing.
     E. Touching the tracheal wall to stimulate a cough.

	Content/ Reinforcement Delivered Date & RN	Learner Objectives Met Date & RN	Not Applicable

V. The patient describes the care of the equipment.
  A. The suction catheter should be changed daily, not necessarily after each suctioning.
  B. The catheter should be kept in a clean towel when not in use.
  C. The collection bottle should be emptied and washed daily.
VI. The patient describes problems that may be encountered related to suctioning.
  A. If secretions can be coughed out, suctioning is not mandatory.
  B. If secretions are thick, suctioning may not clear them and extra humidification may be necessary.
  C. Oversuctioning may cause bleeding or increased secretions.
VII. The patient describes methods to relieve difficult breathing.
  A. Cough and suction.
  B. Remove the inner tube and check to see if it is clear.
  C. Contact the physician if breathing remains difficult.
  D. Go to the nearest emergency room with an extra tube if difficulty is severe.			

Evaluation If patient or significant others are unable to complete some or all of this teaching plan, document evaluation in progress notes.			

GUIDELINES: PATIENT INSTRUCTION FOR TRACHEAL SUCTIONING

I. Purpose

The suction catheter collects secretions from the inner tracheotomy tube. It will stimulate coughing if it touches the tracheal wall. You may suction only to clear the inner tube or purposely to induce coughing. Secretions may occasionally be coughed up orally around the tracheotomy tube.

II. Equipment

Suction machine
Suction catheters
Connecting tubing
Container of water
Cover for suction catheter

III. Use of equipment

Turn on the suction machine, cover the outlet on the catheter with your thumb, and suction some water to make sure that the machine is working. The outlet on the catheter can turn the suction on and off.

IV. Suctioning procedure

Insert the suction catheter into your tracheotomy tube (only the length of the tube), cover the outlet with your thumb, and rotate the catheter as it is withdrawn (use a mirror if possible). It may be helpful to cough first and then suction secretions. Touching the tracheal wall by inserting the suction catheter further than the inner tube will stimulate coughing. This may be done if necessary to remove deep secretions. A small amount of blood tinged secretion may be noticed if the suctioning is too vigorous.

V. Care of equipment

The suction catheter need not be changed with each use but should be rinsed well. A clean catheter should be used every day. The suction catheter should be kept covered between uses (with a clean towel) and the suction bottle should be emptied and washed well daily.

VI. When suctioning is necessary

Suctioning is not mandatory if secretions can be coughed out. If secretions are copious and tend to block the tracheotomy tube, suctioning could be done before cleaning the tracheotomy tube and between cleanings if necessary. Overuse of suctioning may irritate the trachea and cause a small amount of bleeding.

VII. Methods to relieve breathing difficulty

Cough and suction first. Next remove the inner tube and check to make sure it is clear. Humidification should be increased, for example, by sitting directly in front of the vaporizer. If you are still unrelieved, contact your doctor.

If breathing difficulty is acute, go to the nearest emergency room and *bring your duplicate tracheotomy tube with you.*

Physician #: _____

Emergency room #: _____

Part IX

Pediatrics

	Content/ Reinforcement Delivered Date & RN	Learner Objectives Met Date & RN	Not Applicable

PEDIATRIC CARDIAC SURGERY: PREOPERATIVE PREPARATION

Purpose

To retain the child's sense of trust through honest preparation.

To reduce the parents' and child's fear and anxiety through anticipation of events and an understanding of the cardiac defect and its surgical correction.

To help parents provide appropriate emotional support for their child throughout the hospitalization.

To gain cooperation from the parents and child in assisting with the plan of care.

To provide an opportunity for the parents and child to express feelings about hospitalization and cardiac surgery.

Content

   I. Normal heart function
  II. Child's cardiac defect
 III. Surgical correction and coronary bypass
  IV. Preoperative preparation
   V. Anesthesia
  VI. Child's postoperative appearance
 VII. Postoperative environment and routine
VIII. Teaching through role play

Learner Objectives

Child (4 years of age and older)

   I. The child describes to the nurse that the heart is a pump that sends blood to all parts of the body so it can work. (The older child is able to describe, using a diagram, the general heart anatomy and physiology with increasing detail.)
  II. The child says simply that something is wrong with the heart. (The older child is able to describe, or demonstrate on a diagram, the defect and why it needs to be corrected.)
 III. The child describes how the defect will be corrected. (The older child is able to describe the procedure in more detail.)
  IV. The child discusses the events preceding the operation.
   V. The child describes the effect of the anesthetic during the operation.
  VI. The child indicates the site of the incision.
 VII. The child discusses the postoperative routine.
        A. The child relates that parents cannot stay in the intensive care unit but may visit for a short time.
        B. The child demonstrates respiratory care exercises.

	Content/ Reinforcement Delivered Date & RN	Learner Objectives Met Date & RN	Not Applicable
C. The child recognizes the postoperative equipment as it appears on the teaching doll.			
D. The child relates events after the first 24 hours postoperatively.			
VIII. The child takes part in role play with the nurse.			
Parents			
I. The parents describe, using a diagram, the basic anatomy and physiology of the heart.			
II. The parents describe in basic terms their child's defect and cardiac symptoms, if present.			
III. The parents describe in basic terms the surgical procedure to be performed.			
IV. The parents describe the preoperative routine for their child and their participation in it.			
V. The parents describe the effects of the anesthetic during the child's operation.			
VI. The parents indicate the site of the child's incision.			
VII. The parents describe the postoperative routine for their child and their participation in it.			
VIII. The parents discuss their child's possible emotional reaction to cardiac surgery and the measures that can be taken to minimize emotional trauma.			

Evaluation

If patient or significant others are unable to complete some or all of this teaching plan, document evaluation in progress notes.

GUIDELINES: PEDIATRIC CARDIAC SURGERY— PREOPERATIVE PREPARATION

Note for the nurse: A cooperative effort by both floor and intensive care unit nurses is needed to complete this teaching plan.

All parents of children undergoing cardiac surgery are usually well aware of the risks involved. However, parents of an asymptomatic child sometimes have difficulty understanding the real need for corrective surgery. Generally those with a very ill child understand the importance of the operation and the possible risk but also realize that life may be impossible without it. Parents react in many different ways, including guilt, fear, anxiety, denial, despair, hope, and anger. From the beginning, it is necessary to evaluate the parents' understanding of their child's cardiac disease and the surgical procedure. The nurse must also listen to their fears, evaluate their feelings, and determine the external support available through family and friends.

Some parents do not wish their child to receive preoperative instruction; therefore, it must be explained and stressed to them that teaching is necessary for their child to trust staff and thus be less fearful of the operation. The nurse must assure the parents of always being available to help them honestly answer their child's questions and reinforce prior instruction. Sound interviewing techniques and a calm, supportive attitude are necessary.

A child generally does not realize the risks involved in the operation. Often the child does not feel sick at all and may view hospitalization as a punishment. In some cases, the child is too young to understand anything. It is necessary therefore to evaluate each child's potential to understand and to work with each child as an individual. Often the only thing that can be accomplished is gaining the child's trust in the environment and the staff. The child will feel less threatened and be able to understand being loved and cared for even though something will hurt.

Primary nursing is extremely valuable in dealing with a child undergoing cardiac surgery and also in helping parents. This concept enables the parents and child to develop a consistent relationship with one person from the beginning to the end of the hospitalization.

Before initiating teaching, it is important to evaluate both the parents and child in regard to previous hospital experience, parents' knowledge and understanding of the child's illness and need for corrective surgery, level of the parents' understanding, the child's age and level of development and understanding, and available support systems. Any defenses present, such as anxiety, depression, guilt, anger, and denial, must be recognized and dealt with or teaching will be ineffective. Teaching sessions should then be planned according to the nurse's evaluation of the parents and child. Initially they should be taught together, but, later, instruction should be given separately. The teaching should be evaluated for effectiveness by asking questions, encouraging feedback, and giving necessary reinforcement.

For further guidelines refer to the general preoperative teaching of a child and family teaching plan.

I. The child describes to the nurse that the heart is a pump that sends blood to all parts of the body so it can work. (The older child is able to describe, using a diagram, the general heart anatomy and physiology with increasing detail.) Parents describe, using a diagram, the basic anatomy and physiology of the heart.

The nurse describes the anatomy and physiology of the heart, including the four chambers, the valves, and the greater vessels, as well as a simple explanation of the circulatory system. Simple diagrams are available or can be drawn by the nurse.

II. The child says simply that something is wrong with the heart. (The older child is able to describe, or demonstrate on a diagram, the defect and why it needs to be corrected.)

Parents describe in basic terms their child's defect and cardiac symptoms, if present.

The nurse explains the child's defect with the use of diagrams and simple explanations. The nurse incorporates the child's presenting symptoms to enhance understanding. The following are some common defects encountered:

A. Acyanotic
   1. Coarctation of the aorta—a narrowing of the aorta. Symptoms depend on the degree of constriction. This condition often goes unrecognized until late childhood or early adulthood, when the elevation of blood pressure in the arms and low pressure in the legs become evident. With greater constriction comes growth interference, fatigue, weakness in the legs, and congestive heart failure in severe cases.
   2. Aortic stenosis—an obstruction to the flow of blood out of the left ventricle resulting from congenital malformation of the valves, the aortic ring, or the tissue below the valves. In mild cases the child is asymptomatic. If the constriction is severe, fatigue and fainting spells may occur.
   3. Pulmonic stenosis—an obstruction to the outflow of blood from the right ventricle due to an abnormality of the valves of the pulmonic ring. The child may be asymptomatic or with severe stenosis exhibit dyspnea on exertion.
B. Potentially cyanotic
   1. Patient ductus arteriosus—an opening between the descending aorta and the pul-

monary artery, which is present during fetal life and allows blood to bypass the pulmonary system. This usually closes shortly after birth. This condition may interfere with physical activity and growth if the opening is large.

2. Atrial septal defect—an abnormal opening between the right and left atria. Symptoms often seen are slow growth and poor tolerance for exercise. Rheumatic fever and increased susceptibility to pneumonia are associated with this defect.

3. Ventricular septal defect—an abnormal opening between the right and left ventricles. No symptoms occur with small defects located low on the septum and treatment is not usually necessary. Children with larger defects located high on the septum often present with growth impairment, dyspnea, feeding difficulties, and repeated respiratory infections.

C. Cyanotic

1. Tetralogy of Fallot—a combination of a ventricular septal defect, pulmonary stenosis (valvular or infundibular), and an aorta overriding the ventricular septal defect. Children with this defect often have attacks of paroxysmal dyspnea characterized by air hunger, deep cyanosis, and loss of consciousness with or without convulsions. These attacks tend to occur during the first 2 years of life. Children with tetralogy of Fallot often limit their own activity because of fatigue and anoxia. They have a chronic circulatory disturbance to the brain with some degree of anoxia.

2. Tricuspid atresia—no opening exists between the right atrium and the right ventricle. This is incompatible with life unless a ventricular septal defect or a patent ductus arteriosus is present. These infants are cyanotic and without surgical correction often die within a year.

3. Transposition of the great vessels—the aorta originates from the right ventricle; therefore the left side of the heart supplies the pulmonary circuit with oxygenated blood. An abnormal communication (ventricular septal defect, atrial septal defect, or a patent ductus arteriosus) must be present to sustain life. Prognosis is poor without a complicated operation, which has a high mortality rate.

4. Truncus arteriosus—a fusing of the aorta and pulmonary artery causes the entire pulmonary and systemic circulation to be supplied from a common arterial trunk. Cyanosis, dyspnea,

and growth failure occur in varying degrees of severity.

5. Anomalous venous return—oxygenated blood returning from the lungs is carried abnormally by one or more pulmonary veins emptying into the right atrium. Cyanosis, fatigue, and congestive heart failure occur in varying degrees. Total anomalous return occurs when all the pulmonary veins drain into the right side of the circulation, thus depriving the systemic circulation of oxygenated blood. This is incompatible with life unless an atrial septal defect is present to permit some oxygenated blood to return to the left atrium and ventricle. Partial anomalous return occurs when only some of the veins connect with the left atrium.

Other defects or combinations of defects may be seen but are not as common as those just mentioned.

III. The child describes how the defect will be corrected. (The older child is able to describe the procedure in more detail.)

The parents describe in basic terms the surgical procedure to be performed.

The surgical correction should be explained to the child and parents by first explaining the defect and then showing them the site of the repair on the heart diagram. It may be described as "sewing the hole together" or "putting a patch or artificial valve in." Actual patches or valves may be shown.

The heart-lung machine takes over the functions of the heart and lungs during surgical intervention to the heart. Blood is diverted into the machine, which oxygenates the blood and pumps it back into the arterial system by way of the femoral or subclavian artery, thus achieving the functions of the heart and lungs.

IV. The child discusses the events preceding the operation.

Parents describe the preoperative routine for their child and their participation in it.

The next consideration in the preoperative teaching of the child is physical management. Several persons from the medical team visit the patient preoperatively for teaching.

A. The nurse introduces the family and child to the preoperative unit and routine, including blood work, chest x-ray, electrocardiogram, urinalysis, urine culture, nose and throat cultures, antiseptic soap scrubs, and physical examinations by the surgical team and cardiologists.

B. The cardiothoracic surgical team instructs the family about the cardiac disease, the operation itself and its risks, some postoperative details, and possible complications. A permit is then obtained.

C. The chest physiotherapist visits the child and evaluates capacity to participate in chest physiotherapy.

D. On the day of surgery the child is allowed nothing by mouth after midnight. Three injections of prophylactic cefazolin (Kefzol) are administered. The child is brought to the operating room on a stretcher and should be told to expect doctors, nurses, and other operating room personnel dressed in blue hats and masks. The child goes to sleep and on waking in the intensive care unit, the heart is "fixed."

E. The child's parents are told to wait on the unit and just before the final suturing someone from the operating room calls them. The surgeon talks with the parents on the unit to discuss the outcome of the child's operation. As soon as the child is stabilized in the ICU, the parents may visit for 5 minutes, usually with the nurse. The purpose of this visit is to reassure the parents. They are then encouraged to go home and rest. A member of the surgical team telephones late in the evening to give them a final condition report for the night. The parents are told that they may call at any time.

V. The child describes what effect the anesthetic will have during the operation.

Parents describe the effects of the anesthetic during the child's operation.

The anesthesiologist explains the role during the operation and the child's postoperative respiratory care. The child is allowed to choose a scent of anesthetic such as orange or bubble gum.

VI. The child indicates the site of the incision.

The parents indicate the site of the child's incision.

With a teaching doll, the nurse demonstrates where on the child's body the incision will be located, explains that there will be a bandage over the incision, and shows a sample bandage.

VII. The child discusses the postoperative routine.

Parents describe the postoperative routine for their child and their participation in it.

The nurse explains the postoperative routine through the use of a teaching doll, actual equipment, and a coloring book. The child should be allowed to play with the doll and handle the equipment. The child and parents should be encouraged to ask questions and express feelings. The nurse needs feedback from them to evaluate their understanding.

A. The child relates that parents cannot stay in the intensive care unit but may visit for short periods of time. On the day of the operation the patient is taken on a tour of the intensive care unit by the nurses. In the unit the child is shown the equipment and weighed. Reinforce to the patient that a bed in the ICU is a stretcher. The ICU nurses should introduce the child and parents to the unit's environment and personnel. A nurse should demonstrate some of the equipment and their sounds. An explanation of the routines, policies, and visiting regulations is given. The parents may not stay with the child in the ICU, but they should know that they can visit for a few minutes several times a day. Parents are given the ICU telephone number and a booklet describing the unit.

B. The child demonstrates respiratory care exercises. Explain the purpose and use of the triflow device.

C. The child recognizes the postoperative equipment as it appears on the teaching doll.

1. Chest tubes. These tubes drain off air and blood from the chest. They are connected to a plastic container and make a bubbling noise. In a day or two the physician removes the tubes. Little black stitches are used to close the opening and a bandage is placed over them when the chest tube is removed.

2. Nasogastric tube. When the child awakens, there will be a tube in the nose that goes into the stomach. It will keep the stomach empty and prevent the child from getting sick.

3. Endotracheal tube. There will be a tube in the nose or mouth that goes down the trachea. This tube may be attached to a respirator to assist breathing. When the tube is in, the child will not be able to talk. Show the Ambu bag and explain that its purpose is to give deep breaths. Explain what suctioning is and that it is necessary to remove secretions.

4. ECG leads and monitor. Chest wires will be attached to the monitor that will show a picture of the heartbeat on a television screen. In this way the physicians and nurses can watch the heart closely. If appropriate, reinforce that these wires will not electrically shock the child.

5. Intravenous feedings. Because the patient cannot eat for awhile, there will be tubes going into the arms and legs to give fluids and medications. Nurses will also draw blood samples from these tubes, but the child will not feel this. The intravenous setup will be attached to small machines that may beep at times. The legs and arms will be tied down to prevent the disconnection of these tubes.

6. Foley catheter. This will be put in when the patient is sleeping (in the operating room). The tube goes into the bladder to drain the urine into a bag, permitting the child to remain in bed. Use a diagram or doll to demonstrate.

D. The child relates events after the first 24 hours postoperatively.
   1. Tubes will gradually be removed.
   2. The child will have a chest x-ray examination and be weighed every morning.
   3. The child will need to stay in bed for awhile to give the heart a rest. The child will gradually sit up, then ambulate after returning to the floor.
   4. The child will be NPO for awhile; then fluids may be restricted. Diet will gradually be advanced.
   5. The child may find it difficult to sleep in the ICU because of the lights and noise.
   6. The patient will be able to return to the floor once the tubes are removed and the child feels better. It is important not to give a specific time for the patient's return to the floor. It should be emphasized to the parents that the patients are moved out of the ICU as soon as possible, but sometimes the child must wait for an appropriate bed.
   7. The child will gradually progress to ambulating, eating a full diet, and going to the playroom after returning to the floor.

VIII. The child takes part in role play with the nurse.

The parents discuss their child's possible emotional reaction to cardiac surgery and the measures that can be taken to minimize emotional trauma.

Child

Common reactions to an operation are anger, fear, withdrawal, regression, increased dependency, and rejection. The child can be expected to regress after the operation, and the nurses should let the child and parents know that this is acceptable and only temporary. It is necessary to care for a child in such a way that the child does not fear abandonment. This enables the child to regain trust in self-ability to deal with threatening situations. Physical contact and emotional support from parents and team members are needed. Parents should be supported by the staff in their attempts to reassure their child.

During recovery, more demands are placed on the child, who may feel helpless and may despair. The child may become demanding, seeking to restore self-esteem and assert the right of independence. The child will work hard to gain

self-mastery, especially in play, when there is energy for it. Physical debilitation not only prevents the child from actively upholding self-esteem but also weakens defenses against fear. This frightens the child and increases helplessness. Resignation may occur if the nurse and parents do not encourage assertiveness, thus letting the child know that people value and respect the child as a person with a mind of one's own. This helps the child reestablish identity and regain autonomy. The child who has regained physical strength, trust, and autonomy and reestablished identity experiences life more positively.

Parents

Many parents have difficulty relinquishing their overprotectiveness of their child. Time is necessary for them to prove to themselves that their child is now capable of increased activity, learning self-care, and tolerating frustration. The nurse should reinforce this learning by allowing parents to see their child playing without signs of distress. With support from trusted staff members they can conquer their fears and find new satisfactions now that the child is less dependent on them.

Methods of Incorporating Play Therapy with Teaching

The use of hand puppets can be an effective means of preparing a child for an operation. It is also a helpful method of assessing how a child feels about the impending operation. Before initiating a teaching session, assemble all the necessary equipment:

1. Father, mother, nurse, physician, and patient puppets
2. Small stethoscope, syringes, bandages, intravenous sctup, chest tubes
3. Miniature hospital comprised of the various areas of the hospital that the child will be visiting (i.e., ICU, OR, and patient's room)

The nurse can use two methods of initiating play with the puppets, the choice depending on the patient's level of cooperativeness. The first method involves the nurse playing the different characters and the patient playing self. Using the various props, the nurse should set up a situation that the child will encounter during hospitalization. After initiating the play session, the nurse can encourage the child to express feelings and concerns by addressing the patient puppet.

Example 1: Patient Johnny plays himself; the nurse plays the parts of a nurse, physician, mother, and father.
Situation: Johnny is being taught about preoperative medication.
NURSE: Before your operation, Johnny, I will have to give you some medication in the form of a shot to make you sleepy.

The nurse can then turn to the patient's puppet and ask the child what he thinks Johnny's puppet will say to this. This method allows the child to express some concerns in a nonthreatening manner through the puppet.

The nurse, in playing the part of mother, father, or physician, can also provide reassurance of everyone's concern for the patient by explaining situations to the child in the following way:

MOMMY PUPPET: I am going to leave the room while Johnny gets his shot because it hurts me to watch. I know I can't stop the shot because I know it will help Johnny.

The second method can be used for children who are too intimidated or too young to take an active role in the puppet play.

Example 2: The nurse explains the situation to the patient and performs the puppet play while the child observes.

NURSE: Tommy is going for a heart operation. I have to give Tommy his preoperative medication.

NURSE PUPPET: Tommy, I have to give you some medication to make you sleepy for your operation. The medication has to be a shot.

TOMMY PUPPET (played by nurse): Yea, but shots hurt and I don't want one.

NURSE PUPPET: Yes, shots hurt, but only for a few minutes and you can yell and scream all you want. After your shot, you can give me one.

TOMMY PUPPET: Well, all right, if I can give you a shot.

NURSE PUPPET: First I'm going to wash your skin with some smelly stuff called alcohol to get any germs off. [Have patient help you wash Tommy puppet's arm off.] Then I'll take the syringe and give you a shot.

[Have the patient help you give Tommy puppet his shot.]

TOMMY PUPPET: [Screams and cries.]

NURSE PUPPET: I'm sorry, Tommy, I know that hurts. Here's a bandage for your booboo. [Have patient apply bandage to the Tommy puppet's arm.]

TOMMY PUPPET: Oh that really hurt, but now I can give you a shot. [The Tommy puppet then gives the nurse puppet a shot.]

Additional Teaching Resources

1. Staff, such as surgical team, anesthesiologist, and cardiology nurse clinician; other children who have had cardiac surgery; and their parents can be helpful.

2. A Playskool hospital can serve the same purpose of role playing as puppet therapy.

3. A body outline and teaching doll with actual equipment attached are useful in clearing up any misconceptions and castration fantasies of the child concerning postoperative appearance.

4. The Visible Man should be used with older children who have a more detailed knowledge of their anatomy. It is effective with older boys and girls (ages 8 to 15) who would be embarrassed by the use of a teaching doll. You should ask the child to explain the anatomy of the Visible Man's heart and relate it to you in terms of the heart defect. This enables you to determine the level of understanding before the teaching session begins. Allow the child to play the role of nurse or doctor with the Visible Man by attaching intravenous tubes, chest tubes, catheters, etc.

5. Gaughen, J., & Gaughen, R. (1973). *Johnny's journey coloring book*. Boston: American Heart Association. This book can best be used as a summary of teaching. You can assess how much the patient has retained by allowing the child to go through the booklet and relate to you what is happening.

6. Rey, H. A., & Rey, M. (1966). *Curious George goes to the hospital*. Boston: Houghton Mifflin Co. The nurse should use this helpful story presentation with preschoolers.

	Content/ Reinforcement Delivered	Learner Objectives Met	Not Applicable
	Date & RN	Date & RN	

PEDIATRIC DAY SURGERY

(To be used in conjunction with specific day surgery handouts)

Purpose

To decrease parental and child anxiety by giving them an explanation of the planned surgery, procedure, and the preoperative and postoperative care necessary for day surgery.

Content

    I. Normal anatomy and physiology
   II. Abnormal anatomy and physiology
  III. Surgery and procedure
  IV. Preoperative care
   V. Anesthesia
  VI. Postoperative routine
 VII. Discharge plans and home care
VIII. Follow-up

Learner Objectives

    I. Parents and child describe the normal anatomy and physiology of _____ as _____
_____.

   II. Parents and child describe the abnormal anatomy and physiology of _____.

  III. Parents describe surgery and/or procedure as _____
_____
_____.

  IV. Parents describe aspects of preoperative care.
     A. The child may have nothing to eat or drink from midnight the night before surgery and/or procedure until after the procedure.
     B. On the day of surgery and/or procedure the child will have a complete health history and physical performed.
     C. On the day of surgery and/or procedure the child will have a blood test.
     D. The date and time of the child's appointment is _____
_____.

   V. The parents and child state how anesthesia will be given.
     A. The parent and child will be seen by an anesthesiologist.
     B. The child (if old enough) will choose the flavor or smell of anesthetic gas that will be used.
     C. The child (if under 12 months) may receive an injection.

	Content/ Reinforcement Delivered	Learner Objectives Met	Not Applicable
	Date & RN	Date & RN	
D. The child may be sleepy, drowsy, or nauseated when recovering from anesthesia.			
VI. Parents describe postoperative and postprocedure routine.			
A. The child will be in the recovery room for a minimum of 1 hour.			
B. The child's physical condition will be _____.			
C. The child may go home when _____.			
D. The parent may be with the child _____.			
VII. Parents describe home care.			
A. Regular diet may be resumed under the following conditions: _____			
B. The child may resume regular activity at the following time: _____			
C. The child's dressing can be removed or replaced at the following time: _____			
D. The child may bathe or swim when: _____			
E. The child may return to school on _____			
F. The expected side effects of surgery, procedure, or anesthesia are _____			
G. The unexpected side effects and reasons to notify physician are _____			
H. Numbers to call if necessary are			
I. Special instructions specific to the surgery or procedure are _____			
VIII. The parents state the date, time, and place of follow-up.			
Evaluation			
If patient or significant others are unable to complete some or all of this teaching plan, document evaluation in progress notes.			

	Content/ Reinforcement Delivered	Learner Objectives Met	Not Applicable
	Date & RN	Date & RN	

NEWBORN CARE

Purpose

To provide a simple explanation to parents of the proper techniques for feeding and bathing their infant.
To provide parents with information on prevention and treatment of accidents in small children.

Content

  I. Explanation of feeding principles
 II. Explanation of the variety of formulas and when solid food additions should be considered
III. Explanation of safe feeding techniques and reminders
 IV. Demonstration of feeding and bubbling
  V. Explanation of important fundamentals of bathing the baby
 VI. Explanation of the leading accidents during the first year of life
     A. Types
     B. Ways to prevent accidents
     C. Emergency phone numbers

Learner Objectives

After reviewing the explanation of feeding principles and techniques and the fundamentals and procedure about the baby's bath.
  I. The parents relate the feeding principles and describe the difference between a specific feeding schedule versus demand feeding.
 II. The parents state facts about formula varieties and solid food additions:
     A. Amount of formula
     _____
     B. When to add solids
     _____
     C. How to add extra calories to formula (when applicable)
     _____
III. The parents relate facts about safe feeding techniques and reminders:
     A. Feeding: an excellent indicator of how the baby is feeling
     B. Vomiting versus "wet burp"
     C. Disinterest in feeding (infant may be sick)
     D. When to call the physician:
        1. Excessive vomiting
        2. Decrease in volume consumed
        3. Increased irritability or decrease in arousability

	Content/ Reinforcement Delivered Date & RN	Learner Objectives Met Date & RN	Not Applicable

IV. The parents demonstrate safe feeding and bubbling of their infant:
  A. Temperature of formula
  B. Head of baby elevated
  C. Entire nipple full of liquid
  D. Bubbling infant—how often
V. Parents discuss bathing.
  A. The parents relate supplies needed for their baby's bath:
    1. Mild soap and shampoo
    2. Basin or tub
    3. Towel and facecloth
  B. The parents assemble the bath supplies and actually demonstrate the bath.
    1. Cleansing the eyes gently with cotton.
    2. Washing the face without soap.
    3. Washing the neck, chest, back, arms, and legs.
    4. Cleansing the genitals of the female infant from front to back. Retracting and cleansing the uncircumsized male's foreskin.
    5. Observing the baby's mouth for white patches called *thrush*. The physician should be contacted if this is seen.
    6. Using powder or corn starch to keep the baby's buttocks dry and prevent chafing.
VI. The parents discuss accidents during the first year of life.
  A. Parents list accidents:
    1. Falls
    2. Ingestion of poisons and foreign objects
    3. Burns
    4. Drowning
    5. Suffocation
    6. Motor vehicle accidents
  B. The parents relate ways of preventing these accidents:
    1. Falls
      a) Never leave a child alone on a table, couch, or bed.
      b) Always strap the child to a chair or stroller.
      c) Always keep stairways blocked and free of clutter.
    2. Ingestion of poisons and foreign objects
      a) Never leave small objects within the child's reach.
      b) Always check toys for safety; do not let the baby play with loose small objects.
      c) Always keep medicine and poisons out of reach and locked up.			

	Content/ Reinforcement Delivered Date & RN	Learner Objectives Met Date & RN	Not Applicable

d) Remember that babies are oral; everything goes into their mouths.
    e) Always keep ipecac in the medicine closet and ask the physician for instructions for its use.
  3. Burns
    a) Never leave matches or lighters within the baby's reach.
    b) Always check temperature of bath water and food.
    c) Always use back burners of stoves; turn handles of pots and pans in.
  4. Drownings. Never leave a child alone in a tub or near lakes, swimming pools, or beaches.
  5. Suffocation
    a) Never leave plastic bags within the baby's reach.
    b) Never use plastic pillow or mattress covers.
    c) Never tie a child to the bed or use stringed clothing.
  6. Motor vehicle accidents
    a) Never leave the child unattended in a car.
    b) Always use car seats and seat belts.
C. The parents state emergency phone numbers:
  1. Fire #: _____
  2. Police #: _____
  3. Physician #: _____
  4. Poison center #: _____		

Evaluation If patient or significant others are unable to complete some or all of this teaching plan, document evaluation in progress notes.		

GUIDELINES: NEWBORN CARE

This teaching plan is designed to provide a simple explanation of proper techniques to parents in the feeding and bathing of their infant. Many first parents are both frightened and anxious to take their baby home. The best we may provide for them is to make sure that they feel comfortable when they are taking their newborn home.

I. The parents relate principles of feeding their baby. It is essential first to explain the feeding principles. Feeding times are one of the most important periods of closeness and contact during the infant's first few months of life. The combination of relief from hunger and being held in a parent's arms establishes contentment for the infant. The parents relate the difference between a feeding schedule versus demand feeding.

 The infant who has been cared for in a hospital nursery has often been on a feeding schedule. It is important to give the parents that schedule so that they will feel comfortable knowing when to feed the baby. Describe to the parents that their baby will eventually advance to less frequent feedings. Explain to them that they may also decide to feed the infant on demand.

II. The parents relate facts about formula varieties and solid food additions.

 Review the formula that the baby has been given in the hospital. Many varieties of a single formula exist in different preparatory forms (e.g., powder), and it would be beneficial for the nurse to be familiar with these. Make sure that the parents understand what to add for extra calories (e.g., corn oil, Karo syrup, etc.). Advise parents to consult their pediatrician about when solid food should be added. Be specific as to how much formula their baby needs to take every feeding. Explain that as the baby grows, it will probably take more formula less often. Ask the doctor for specific formula additives.

III. The parents relate facts about safe feeding techniques and reminders. Each infant is unique. If the parents have any questions as to whether the baby is taking too little or too much, tell them to consult the pediatrician. Remind parents that babies often spit with bubbling. This will be a small amount of formula (5 to 10 cc) referred to as a "wet burp." Try to help distinguish this from vomiting (describe projectile vomiting).

 Feeding is an excellent indicator of how the baby is feeling. A sense for the baby's well-being will come with time. If an infant suddenly or often seems disinterested in feeding, the baby may be feeling sick. Tell the parents to consult the pediatrician if the baby is acting differently during feeding times.

IV. The parents demonstrate safe feeding and bubbling of the infant. The technique of bottle feeding the infant is as follows:
1. Warm the bottle to room temperature or slightly warmer to prevent colic and gas.
2. Cradle the baby in one arm keeping the head well elevated.
3. Keep the bottle tilted so that the entire nipple is full of liquid (this will prevent swallowing of air).
4. Burp the baby frequently—after approximately every ounce to ounce and a half. The baby may be bubbled while being held over the shoulder or sitting the baby in the feeder's lap, supporting the infant with one hand being careful to lean the baby slightly forward.

V. A. The parents relate preparations for their baby's bath. The baby's bath time gives the parents a time to cleanse, play, touch, and observe their child. This is very important to the baby's physical and emotional development. Important points to make to parents are as follows:
1. The baby should be cleansed daily but it does not have to be an immersible bath; it may be a sponge bath.
2. The baby should not have a tub bath until the umbilical cord has fallen off and healed. Wiping the cord stump with isopropyl alcohol with each diaper change will facilitate healing.
3. A parent should *never* leave a child unattended in a tub or on a bathing table.

 Supplies needed for the bath are as follows: mild soap and shampoo, basin or tub, towel, and facecloth. Water temperature must be tepid—warm to elbow touch.
B. The parents assemble the bath supplies and demonstrate the bath. The baby should be bathed beginning at the head and working toward the feet.
1. Cleanse the baby's eyes with cotton balls, one for each eye, wiping from the nose outward. If a parent notices any yellow drainage, a physician should be contacted.
2. The face should be washed with a wet facecloth without soap. Hair should be washed once or twice a week. Parents may be instructed to check the scalp for a yellowish, greasy crust called *cradle cap*. They may also be instructed to warm mineral oil and apply it to the scalp. The oil should be left on 20 to 30 minutes and then the hair should be combed with a fine tooth comb.

3. Next wash the neck, chest, back, arms, legs being careful to clean between all skin folds. If the umbilical cord is still attached, the parents may dab it with isopropyl alcohol at bath time and diaper changes.
4. Genitals of females are always cleansed from front to back. The uncircumcised male should have his foreskin retracted and cleansed daily.
5. The baby's mouth should be observed for white patches called *thrush*. The physician should be contacted if this is seen.
6. Powder or corn starch is helpful in keeping the baby's buttocks dry and to prevent chafing.

VI. A. The parents relate accidents during first year of life.
B. The parents relate ways of preventing these accidents.

We have included a section on accident prevention in this teaching plan because accidents are the leading cause of death in children. It should be part of normal newborn teaching especially with new parents.

The following is a list of ways to assist in preventing the most common accidents during the first year of life.
1. Falls
   a) Never leave a child alone on a table, couch, or bed.
   b) Always strap the child to a chair or stroller.
   c) Always keep stairways blocked and free of clutter.
2. Ingestion of poisons and foreign objects
   a) Never leave small objects within the child's reach.
   b) Always check all toys for safety—no loose small objects.
   c) Always keep medicine and poisons out of reach and locked up.
   d) Remember that babies are oral; everything goes into their mouths.
   e) Always keep ipecac in the medicine closet; ask the physician for instructions.
3. Burns
   a) Never leave matches or lighter within the child's reach.
   b) Always check the temperature of the bath water and food.
   c) Always use the back burners of stoves; turn handles of pots and pans toward the back.
4. Drownings. Never leave a child alone in a tub or near lakes, swimming pools, or beaches.
5. Suffocation
   a) Never leave plastic bags within the child's reach.
   b) Never use plastic pillow or mattress covers.
   c) Never tie a child to a bed or use stringed clothing.
6. Motor vehicle accidents
   a) Never leave a child unattended in a car.
   b) Always use a car seat and seat belts.
C. The parents state emergency phone numbers. If accidents occur, remain calm and always have emergency phone numbers by the telephone (e.g., fire, police, doctor, poison center). Always leave places and numbers to be contacted for babysitters. Call and check with sitters at night.

	Content/ Reinforcement Delivered	Learner Objectives Met	Not Applicable
	Date & RN	Date & RN	

GENERAL PREOPERATIVE TEACHING OF A CHILD AND FAMILY

Purpose

To reduce the parents' and child's fear and anxiety through anticipation of events and an understanding of the surgical procedure. To help parents provide appropriate emotional support for their child throughout the hospitalization.

Content

    I. Reason for the child's hospitalization
   II. Reason for surgery and explanation of the anatomical surgery
  III. Explanation of events immediately surrounding surgery
  IV. Feelings about illness or hospitalization
   V. Reasons for surgery
  VI. Description of operation events

Learner Objectives

    I. Child verbalizes, or expresses through play activities, feelings produced by illness or hospitalization.
   II. Child verbalizes why and where the operation is going to be performed.
  III. Child verbalizes the order in which the major events surrounding the operation will occur and basically describes each event.
  IV. Parents or appropriate family member verbalizes feelings about their child's illness or hospitalization.
   V. Parents or appropriate family member verbalizes why an operation is going to be performed on their child and what it will entail.
  VI. Parents or appropriate family member verbalizes the order in which major events surrounding the operation will occur and gives a basic description of each event.

Evaluation

If patient or significant others are unable to complete some or all of this teaching plan, document evaluation in progress notes.

GUIDELINES: PREOPERATIVE TEACHING OF A CHILD AND FAMILY

Purpose (Why do we do preoperative teaching?)

"It is an all too common practice for parents to tell a child nothing . . . (or to deliver him to the hospital on some pretext) and then abandon him in an atmosphere which is foreign, exciting, and mysterious" (Gross, 1964, p. 8). This can seriously harm the child's ability to trust parents. When a child enters the hospital, many new experiences and frightening situations are encountered. "The child faces a great unknown: cooperation may become impossible. The worries and nightmares which often follow such a profound and terrifying experience can produce lasting mental distortions" (Gross, 1964, p. 8). Thorough preparation preceding each new experience can reduce the child's fears and anxiety. Surgery can be a particularly threatening situation for a child. Preoperative teaching can convey information that will help the child cope with stress. It is not enough to be told a fact once or twice; it must be assimilated. To understand something unknown and fearful, a child needs opportunities to mobilize defenses in order to cope with the situation.

To retain the child's sense of trust, intitiate cooperation, and prevent emotional trauma, the child should be as thoroughly prepared as possible for all procedures, especially surgery. The preoperative teaching can be done by all who care for the child, including the parents, nurses, and physicians. Perhaps the parents have begun to prepare their child for admission and surgery before the child is admitted. This should enhance the teaching done in the hospital. However, whether or not the child has already received information, the child and parents need an opportunity to review the teaching material and to express their fears. The nurses need an opportunity to uncover any misconceptions or fantasies, as well as an opportunity to provide information that will help the child and family cope with the surgical experience.

Teaching Process

The following information is needed before preoperative teaching can be started.

1. An understanding of the principles of learning. How do children learn? What are the obstacles to learning? How do we know if teaching is effective?
   a) Learning is multidimensional. (The child responds as a total individual to the total situation.)
   b) Learning is individual and social. (The child has a unique background.)
   c) Learning is an active process. (The child should be active in learning.)
   d) Learning is purposeful. (The child and teacher should have goals to work toward.)
   e) Learning is creative. (Learning is different for each patient.)
   f) Learning is transferable. (Information learned in one situation applies in another context.)
2. An understanding of the normal growth and development of children, including physical, intellectual, emotional, and social development. What fears are common for this group? What is the child's ability to comprehend? How will the child learn best?
3. An understanding of the operation. What is the child's or family's understanding of what will be done during the operation?
   a) A nurse should accompany the child to the operating room and should be familiar with what is experienced.
   b) Know what the general routine is.
   c) Know what the usual postoperative course is. This takes experience. Sometimes it is not possible to be very specific because the extent of the surgery is unknown. The nurse should not lie but admit to the child the inability to answer specific questions.
   d) Understand the anesthetic method, whether general (mask or intravenous) or local.
4. An understanding of the individual child and family.
   a) What previous experiences have they had affecting this hospitalization?
   b) What is the parents' knowledge of the operation? What have the parents told the child? What do they want the child to know?
   c) What is the child's knowledge of the operation before teaching? Where was the information obtained? What are the child's misconceptions and fantasies?
   d) What support can the family give?
   e) What is the child's developmental level emotionally and intellectually?
   f) What factors may interfere with learning (anxiety, retardation, etc.)?

Fear is not necessarily diminished if a child has had surgery. We often neglect children who have had surgery. They may be the ones most in need of help to express their feelings and their fears and therefore need reassurance. Also, remember that well-educated parents or parents who are medical professionals may need help in preparing for their child's operation.

Teaching Techniques

1. First, the child needs to know, trust, and believe in a person. It is best to get to know the child (e.g., play with the child) before teaching is initiated. If possible, the primary nurse, who knows the child and family best, should do the preoperative teaching.
2. It usually is preferable to do the teaching with the parents present (however, not with adolescents).

3. Begin teaching when the child is ready (within realistic time limits), when there is a relatively calm atmosphere, and not after painful procedures. Do not wait, however, for the child to ask about the operation. The child may be denying surgery and needs the subject brought up.
4. Teach in a nondistracting environment (no television, visitors, children playing noisily). Teach in a nonthreatening place where the child seems relatively secure (e.g., room with personal belongings).
5. Take time to individualize the teaching. Gear the method and information to the child's age, responses, and interest. Get feedback. The child may not be understanding what you say. Ask the child to repeat; insist on involvement.
6. If obstacles arise, defer some teaching until later (e.g., if anxiety is too great or attention span is too short). The preoperative teaching plan allows the nurse to begin teaching whenever the child seems receptive, stop when appropriate, record what was covered, and resume teaching later, even by another individual. Children often need things repeated and time to think over what they were told. Make sure that they do not receive conflicting information. The teaching plan also helps the nurse to be aware of problem areas that others have discovered in talking to the child. What does the child fear most? How can the experience be made easier? What areas need to be reinforced?
7. Be sincere; do not lie or try to cover up facts. Often children ask many questions. If you are unsure of the answers, do not make up anything. You may want to delay or omit areas that you believe the child may not be able to comprehend or cope with; but if a child asks a direct question, you must investigate what the child wishes to know and then get the answers. If you follow the child's cues, you are safe. Too much information may be dangerous; but if you are guided by the child's needs, worries, etc., you usually can judge what to discuss.

Teaching Tools and Resources

Children learn through their senses: visual, auditory, and tactile.

1. Preoperative teaching plan to record information covered in teaching sessions, plus the child's or parents' reactions
2. Masks, gowns, and caps (if age-appropriate)
3. Dolls with bandages, intravenous setups, and casts (as appropriate)
4. Hospital doll house with miniature equipment (if age-appropriate)
5. Apparatus such as anesthesia masks, ECG leads, oxygen cannulas, ileal loop appliances, Foley catheters, Hemovac, and restraints (any equipment a child will be aware of)
6. The Visible Man or anatomical drawings (if age-appropriate)
7. Tour of recovery room and intensive care unit

Content

I/IV. Child verbalizes, or expresses through play activities, feelings produced by illness or hospitalization. Parents or appropriate family member verbalizes feelings about child's illness or hospitalization. Not all the nurse tells the child is future unpleasantness. The nurse can give reassurance that sedatives and anesthetics are worth their discomfort because they will relieve the pain of the operation itself. Offer reassurance as much as possible, but do not forget to warn of the unpleasant experiences (parents often forget to do this). Essential preparation is learning about things that seem dangerous to the child. This is where fantasies and fears arise. Fears of castration, mutilation, and loss of control under anesthesia are common (see Exhibit 2). The child needs to be told about the sensations that will be experienced, people who will be met, and what is expected of the child as a patient.

II/V. Child verbalizes why and where the operation will be performed.
Parents or appropriate family member verbalizes why the operation is going to be performed and what it entails.
Explain the operation and why it is being done (age-appropriate explanations) (Petrillo & Sanger, 1972). A drawing of anatomy and body parts may be helpful. You may want to give the parents a more in-depth explanation either before or after teaching the child.

III/VI. Child verbalizes the order in which the major events surrounding the operation occur and basically describes each event.
Parents or appropriate family member verbalizes the order in which major events surrounding the operation occur and give a basic description of each event. It may be helpful to follow the procedures in chronological order as they happen to the child, but this is not always necessary. Also, the nurse does not need to cover all the material. The teaching must be individualized. The nurse must be receptive to the child's cues and follow the child's speed, according to needs and concerns.

Exhibit 2 Developmental Guidelines for Preoperative Preparation

Age	Cognitive/Emotional Development	Suggestions for Techniques To Diminish Anxiety
Birth to 1 year	Is dependent on mother Satisfaction of basic needs (e.g., warmth, comfort, nourishment, and stimulation) leads to development of trust	Promote healthy infant-family relationship (involve parents in planning and providing care for child) Provide consistent care (mother surrogate), especially in absence of mother or father Explain procedures, operation, etc., to parents and provide emotional support for family members Provide physical comforts and environmental stimulation Comfort child after painful procedure
1 to 3 years	Relationship with parents intense; separation anxiety occurs in their absence Develops trusting relationships Asserts some independence—actively explores world around him Is concerned about body integrity—increased awareness of body Daily routines important to child's sense of security Lacks abstract thought—has poor sense of time	Help parents understand child's reactions following separation from parents Encourage parents to room-in during hospitalization Provide consistent nursing care, especially in absence of parents, comforting child after painful or frightening experiences Be truthful in explanations and keep promises Allow child some degree of independence and control Provide simple explanations about illness or diagnosis Incorporate familiar objects and routines into nursing care Inform child of procedures just before time they are to be performed rather than in advance Postoperatively, show child the dressings and incision and reassure the child that nothing has been removed without knowledge Allow child to express feelings by reenacting procedures on doll or favorite stuffed animal
3 to 7 years	Is interested in roles, especially parental roles Has increased awareness of environment Is able to understand concrete ideas and relationships Maintenance of parental and sibling relationships important Fears abandonment and punishment Has fears and fantasies about real or imagined threats related to body integrity (e.g., castration and mutilation) Is not always able to express feelings verbally	Explain different roles of hospital staff Orient child to room, nursing unit, and other areas of hospital Using diagrams and pictures, explain the child's diagnosis and procedures that are to be performed Encourage parents to visit frequently Explain why the illness has occurred and reassure child that it is not punishment Reassure child that only portion of body described as needing surgical intervention will be operated on—no additional part will be involved Use play therapy to help child act out feelings
7 to 13 years	Is able to reason and make generalizations Understands concept of time Is more able to tolerate separation from parents Peer relationships gain increasing importance Develops ego strengths—fears loss of control Displays increasing self-responsibility Has fear of death	Explain procedures and operations in detail several times in advance; use of Visible Man may be helpful when explaining anatomy Judge how much and when to teach according to child's questions Play interviews may be helpful; provide opportunity for child to interact with other children of same age Be supportive if regressive behaviors appear and help child master those responsibilities capable of assuming Encourage self-care when reasonable

Exhibit 2 continued

Age	Cognitive/Emotional Development	Suggestions for Techniques To Diminish Anxiety
13 to 18 years	Is capable of abstract thinking Shows normal hostility towards parents and questioning of authority figures Emerging identity develops and sense of self Body image very important—is concerned about physical appearance Peer relationships of utmost importance Has fear of dependency	Give thorough explanations of diagnosis and procedures or surgery to be performed Provide opportunity to discuss feelings about hospitalization and illness without parents being present Reassure patient that questions and discussions are confidential Respect need for privacy Be supportive and sensitive to patient's need to cope with temporary or permanent changes in physical appearance and capabilities Provide opportunity for continuation of social relationships Allow as much independence as possible

A. NPO. What it means. Why must the child be NPO?

B. Preoperative medication. If a younger child is to get an injection, it may be helpful to defer this aspect of teaching until later. The young child may focus on this area only and not listen to the remainder of the teaching. Explain why the medication is given and what will happen. The child will feel drowsy and have a dry mouth.

C. Trip to operating room. Preferably the child is escorted to the operating room by the primary nurse or another staff member. The child will ride on a stretcher or in a go-cart. Describe the operating room: people's dress, odors, equipment such as the operating table, lights, and the cooled air. Explain that there will probably be a wait in the hall until the physicians are ready.

D. Anesthesia. If the type of anesthesia is not known, mention both intravenous injection and mask (have a younger child handle the mask). Describe the various smells or "flavors" of anesthetic agents. Explain to the child that "a special doctor (anesthetist) will give you medicine to make you sleep while the doctor fixes your _____, and you will be awakened when the operation is all over." (Fear of never waking up or fear of waking up in the middle of the operation is common.) For a younger child do not include any details of the surgery itself, since the child will not be awake during the operation (no mention of cutting should be made). Describe what the child will find after waking.

E. Recovery room. (If going to intensive care unit, explain at this time; see pediatric cardiac surgery teaching plan.) Explain to the child about awakening in a small room where there are other patients who have had operations. A special nurse will be watching and will take vital signs. Mention that frequent taking of vital signs is routine—it may frighten the older child. Explain the use of restraints, mention deep breathing and coughing, and discuss other treatments that will be performed. Also explain that intravenous equipment, tubes, and dressings may be in place. Describe their purpose, approximately how long they will be used, and their disposition after use.

F. Return to room. Explain to the child that when fully awake, the child will be returned to the room and someone will be waiting (nurse and possibly parents). The child will be returned to own bed. A nurse will check often. If appropriate, mention the following:

1. At the proper time the child will be told when to eat and to get out of bed.

2. If discomfort or pain occurs, medication can be given to alleviate it.

3. It is important to turn, cough, and deep breathe. Practice this preoperatively. (Use appropriate equipment.)

4. The use of bedpans or urinals may be necessary.

Evaluation

The child's postoperative course will reflect the preoperative teaching that has been received. Is there some degree of trust in parents and hospital staff? Within reason, does the child cooperate with the postoperative treatments and restrictions? Is there free expression of feelings about the operation and hospitalization? Does the child (within the structure of individual personality) adjust to the hospital experience without any major behavioral disorders?

Preoperative teaching of children may have varying degrees of success; the same teaching preparation may produce different results in different children. "We must not think that any child who has been properly prepared will go into surgery like a lamb while an unprepared child will not" (Plank et al., 1971, p. 22). The opposite may be true. The child who has not received adequate preoperative teaching will not know what to expect and thus may show little outward anxiety or may be very docile. However, the postoperative adjustment period may be emotionally traumatic for this child. "The value of good preparation for an operation appears afterwards, in the speed of recuperation and in freedom from neurotic symptoms" (Plank et al., 1971, p. 22).

BIBLIOGRAPHY

Bergmann, T., in collaboration with A. Freud. (1965). *Children in the hospital*. New York: International Universities Press, Inc.

Gross, R.E. (1964). *The surgery of infancy and children*. Philadelphia: W.B. Saunders Co.

Haller, J.A. (1967). *The hospitalized child and his family*. Baltimore: Johns Hopkins University Press.

Hardgrove, C.G., & Dawson, R.B. (1972). *Parents and children in the hospital*. Boston: Little, Brown & Co.

Inhelder, B., & Piaget, J. (1958). *The growth of logical thinking from childhood to adolescence*. New York: Basic Books.

Petrillo, M. (1968). Preventing hospital trauma in pediatric patients. *American Journal of Nursing, 68*:1468–1473.

Petrillo, M., & Sanger, S. (1972). *Emotional care of hospitalized children*. Philadelphia: J.B. Lippincott Co.

Plank, E.N., et al. (1971). *Working with children in hospitals* (2nd ed.). Cleveland: Yearbook Medical Publishers.

Prugh, D.G., et al. (1953). A study of emotional reactions of children and families to hospitalization and illness. *American Journal of Orthopsychiatry, 23*:70–106.

Scahill, M. (1969, June). Preparing children for procedures and operations. *Nursing Outlook, 17*:36–38.

Scipien, G.M., et al. (1975). *Comprehensive pediatric nursing*. New York: McGraw-Hill Book Co.

Vaughan, V.C., & McKay, R.J. (Eds.). (1975). *Nelson textbook of pediatrics* (10th ed.). Philadelphia: W.B. Saunders Co.

Vernon, D.T.A., et al. (1965). *The psychological responses of children to hospitalization and illness: A review of the literature*. Springfield, Ill.: Charles C. Thomas, Pub.

Waechter, E.H., & Blake, D.G. (1976). *Nursing care of children* (9th ed.). Philadelphia: J.B. Lippincott Co.

Part X

Medication

	Content/ Reinforcement Delivered Date & RN	Learner Objectives Met Date & RN	Not Applicable

MEDICATION

Purpose

To facilitate compliance with the medication regimen.

Content

    I. Drug description
       A. Name
       B. Classification
       C. Appearance
   II. Reasons for prescription
 III. Proper use of medication
       A. Dosage
       B. Time
       C. Special considerations
  IV. Side effects
       A. Common—nonreportable
       B. Reportable
   V. Reasons to notify physician
       A. Problem with medication schedule
       B. Side effects
       C. New prescription
       D. Physician
  VI. Handout

Learner Objectives

    I. The patient states description of drug in the following terms:
       A. Name of drug is _____
       B. Drug category is _____
       _____
       C. Drug looks like _____
       _____

   II. The patient states the reason for taking the drug: _____

 III. The patient states the proper use of medication in the following terms:
       A. Correct dosage is _____
       _____
       B. Correct medication schedule is _____
       _____

	Content/ Reinforcement Delivered Date & RN	Learner Objectives Met Date & RN	Not Applicable

C. Special considerations in taking this drug are (i.e., full stomach; interaction with other drugs; take with milk) _____ _____ _____
 	
IV. The patient describes side effects of the medication in the following terms:
   A. 5 most common side effects that *do not* need to be reported to the physician:
     1. _____
     2. _____
     3. _____
     4. _____
     5. _____
   B. Side effects that *must be* reported to the physician:
_____ _____ _____ _____ _____
 	
V. The patient describes the following as reasons to notify the physician:
   A. Inability to maintain medication schedule
   B. Appearance of any of the above side effects that *must be* reported to the physician
   C. Need for new prescription
   D. Physician's number: _____
VI. The patient takes medication handout home.
 	
Evaluation
 	
If patient or significant others are unable to complete some or all of this teaching plan, document evaluation in progress notes.		

	Content/ Reinforcement Delivered Date & RN	Learner Objectives Met Date & RN	Not Applicable

CORTICOSTEROID REPLACEMENT THERAPY
 	
Purpose
 	
To teach the person dependent on replacement corticosteroids the physiologic mechanism and the importance of replacement treatment, side effects, toxicity, and what to do in situations of acute stress.
 	
Content
 	
   I. Individual reason for steroid treatment
  II. The drugs and their particular properties
 III. Administration
 IV. Normal side effects
  V. Reasons to contact the physician
 VI. Prevention of problems
 	
Learner Objectives
 	
   I. The patient explains the reason for steroid treatment.			

II. The patient names the medication and describes its use and correct dosage.			
III. The patient describes the drug that will be taken and develops an appropriate dosage schedule.			
IV. The patient lists normal side effects caused by steroid medication.			

	Content/ Reinforcement Delivered Date & RN	Learner Objectives Met Date & RN	Not Applicable
V. The patient describes when and how to notify the physician.			
VI. The patient describes ways of preventing problems.			
Evaluation If the patient or significant others are unable to complete some or all of this teaching plan, document evaluation in progress notes.			

GUIDELINES: CORTICOSTEROID
REPLACEMENT THERAPY

Background for the nurse: One of the uses of corticosteroid drugs is as a replacement medication for those persons whose adrenal cortex does not produce adequate corticosteroids. The secretion of corticosteroids (or adrenocortical hormones) from the adrenal cortex is regulated by the release of adrenocorticotrophic hormone (ACTH from the anterior pituitary gland). ACTH is in turn secreted in response to a releasing factor from the hypothalamus of the brain and regulated by a feedback loop.

Adrenocortical hormones are classified as (1) mineralocorticoids, (2) glucocorticoids, and (3) androgenic hormones. The first two are essential for survival.

Mineralocorticoids (aldosterone) are important in regulating salt and water metabolism and electrolyte balance. Lack of aldosterone can cause shocklike symptoms, leading to circulatory collapse and ultimately coma and death.

Glucocorticoids (cortisol and hydrocortisone) have extremely important and complex regulatory functions, including effects on carbohydrate, protein, and fat metabolism; inhibition of inflammatory and allergic response; and rapid and efficient mobilization of energy resources in response to stress.

The corticosteroids must be compensated for if the adrenal cortex fails to synthesize adequate amounts. Some patients are only mildly insufficient in corticosteroids and get along well ordinarily, showing symptoms only when subjected to unusual stress. Others have a complete lack of cortical hormones and are totally dependent on receiving substitution therapy. Adrenal insufficiency can be caused by a variety of conditions:

1. Addison's disease (atrophy of the adrenal gland from idiopathic causes)
2. Adrenalectomy (for pheochromocytoma, carcinoma, etc.)
3. Hypophysectomy (for pituitary adenoma)
4. Hypopituitarism
5. Hypothalamic dysfunction
6. Adrenal atrophy from overuse of glucocorticoids or ACTH

Replacement therapy is given in large dosages during stress or crisis and in small dosages for maintenance.

I. The patient explains the personal reason for steroid treatment.
Explain to the patient: Your body is not making enough of a certain hormone called *cortisol.* You must have this hormone to live; therefore, to get the amount of this hormone needed, you must take steroid medication every day.

This hormone is used by the body in several ways. It has an important role in the breakdown and use of sugars, starches, protein, and fat found in the food that you eat. It also prevents inflammation and is extremely important in helping the body recover after stress.

II. The patient names the medication and describes its use and correct dosage.
Explain to the patient: There are many different kinds of steroid drugs. They each can replace the hormone that your body cannot produce; however, some are stronger than others or act a little differently. Your physician will tell you which one is best for you.
For the nurse: The most common pill forms follow:

Generic names	Brand names
Cortisone	Cortogen, Cortone
Dexamethasone	Decadron, Hexadrol
Fludrocortisone	Florinef (used only if both adrenal glands have been removed)
Prednisolone	
Prednisone	
Triamcinolone	Aristocort, Kenacort

The injectable drugs that patients might be advised to keep follow:

Generic names	Brand names
Cortisone	
Dexamethasone	Decadron
Hydrocortisone	Solu-Cortef
Methylprednisolone	Solu-Medrol

If the patient cannot remember the drug's specific name, it is important that the person at least describe the medication as a steroid pill or injection.

III. The patient describes how to take the drug and develops the most appropriate schedule.
Explain to the patient: To avoid irritating the stomach, steroid medication should be taken with milk or antacids or after meals. Since the pills must be taken at the same time every day, you should decide on the time of day that is most convenient for you. Oral medication is best taken on waking in the morning. If there are two doses, the second dose should be taken in the late afternoon. Intramuscular injections should be taken in the morning. An index card showing the medication schedule may be posted where it is easily seen to remind you to take your medication.

IV. The patient lists normal side effects caused by steroid medication.
Explain to the patient: Some possible changes should not alarm you. These include the following:
1. Slight weight gain caused by the retention of salt and water in the body. This can be minimized by using less salt with the food that you eat.
2. Stomach upset after taking the medication.

3. Changes in mood.

4. Changes in pattern of menstruation.

V. The patient describes when and how to notify the physician.

Explain to the patient: The following problems may occur:

1. Swelling of the ankles, face, or belly; excessive weight gain.

2. Pain in the chest or legs.

3. Bleeding from the mouth or blood in the stool.

4. Persistent stomach pain or indigestion.

5. Signs of crises:
   a. Nausea, diarrhea
   b. Severe headache or trouble with vision
   c. Weakness, dizziness, or unusual fatigue

6. Signs of stress. Stress is anything that unexpectedly makes you work harder, either physically or mentally. Examples follow:
   a. Accidents
   b. Infections
   c. Influenza or colds
   d. Intense heat or cold
   e. Depression, loss of a loved one, or loss of a job
   f. Any major change in normal lifestyle

Call the physician immediately for these stressful circumstances. If you are unable to make contact, go to the nearest emergency room.

Note for the nurse: The nurse should help the patient identify the stresses in day-to-day living and working environment.

VI. The patient describes ways of preventing problems.

Explain to the patient:

1. Take the correct amount of the steroid medication at the same time every day. Never skip a dose; never stop taking the drug.

2. Notify the physician immediately when signs of crisis or circumstances of stress occur.

3. Schedule regular examinations with your physician.

4. Inform all health providers—physicians, dentists, and optometrists—who care for you that you are taking steroid medication.

5. Wear a medic alert tag or bracelet so that others will be aware of the need for steroid medication, especially in case of an emergency.

	Content/ Reinforcement Delivered Date & RN	Learner Objectives Met Date & RN	Not Applicable

DIGOXIN ADMINISTRATION FOR THE PEDIATRIC PATIENT
 	
Purpose
 	
To facilitate compliance with digoxin administration.
To educate the patient and family about the action, administration, and possible side effects of digoxin.
 	
Content
 	
I. Description of digoxin
II. Reasons for the prescription
III. Proper use of digoxin
IV. Side effects
V. Signs of congestive heart failure
VI. Safety measures
VII. Reasons to notify the physician
VIII. Handout
 	
Learner Objectives
 	
I. The patient and parents describe digoxin.
  A. The name of the drug is *digoxin*.
  B. Digoxin improves the strength and efficiency of the heart.
  C. The patient's digoxin dose appears as
    1. Elixir containing 0.05 mg/cc.
    2. Yellow unscored tablets of 0.125 mg.
    3. White scored tablets of 0.25 mg.
    4. Green scored tablets of 0.5 mg.
II. The patient and parents state that digoxin is used to help to control congestive heart failure or to control the rate of the heart beat.
III. The patient and parents state the proper use of digoxin in the following terms:
  A. The correct dosage is _____.
  B. The correct medication schedule is _____.
  C. If the child vomits the entire dose within minutes after taking it, repeat the dose one time.
  D. The patient and parents demonstrate the proper procedure of administration of digoxin elixir.
  E. If digoxin is used to control tachyarrhythmias, the patient and parents demonstrate the ability to take an apical pulse for 1 minute.			

	Content/ Reinforcement Delivered	Learner Objectives Met	Not Applicable
	Date & RN	Date & RN	

IV. The patient and parents state side effects of digoxin:
  A. Increased vomiting or onset of vomiting in a child who does not usually vomit
  B. Poor feeding in an infant; marked decrease in appetite in an older child
  C. Nausea in an older child
  D. Increased irritability or restlessness
  E. Fatigue, especially in an older child
  F. Changes in electrocardiogram pattern
V. The patient and parents state signs of congestive heart failure:
  A. Increased respiratory rate or labored respirations, especially when the child is asleep
  B. Increased shortness of breath with activity and feeding
  C. Increased sweating, especially when feeding
  D. Frequency of urination and amount of urine decreased by half
  E. Edema, especially of extremities, perineal or scrotal area, or, in infants, around the eyes
  F. Increased irritability or restlessness
  G. Increased fatigue with normal activity
  H. Cool temperature
VI. The patient and parents state safety measures to be followed.
  A. Digoxin must be kept out of the reach of children.
  B. If the elixir is used, a spare bottle should be kept at home.
  C. Ipecac should be kept at home in case of accidental overdose.
VII. The patient and parents describe the following as reasons to notify physician:
  A. Inability to maintain the medication schedule
  B. Appearance of side effects
  C. Signs of increasing congestive heart failure
  D. Need for a new prescription
  E. Physician's telephone #: _____
VIII. The patient and parents take the handout home.
 	
Evaluation
 	
If patient or significant others are unable to complete some or all of this teaching plan, document evaluation in progress notes.			

	Content/ Reinforcement Delivered Date & RN	Learner Objectives Met Date & RN	Not Applicable
WARFARIN (COUMADIN) **Purpose** To provide the patient with a basic understanding of the action of warfarin and the necessary precautions that should be observed by individuals taking this medication. **Content** I. An explanation of the action of warfarin and its use II. Discussion of dosage and administration of the drug III. Discussion of side effects IV. Special teaching needs in regard to warfarin V. Review of warfarin booklet			
Learner Objectives I. The patient explains why warfarin has been prescribed and what effect it has on clotting.			
II. The patient states the following with regard to the use of warfarin: A. Dosage of the drug			
B. Frequency of administration and what to do if a dose is missed			
C. Storage of the drug			

	Content/ Reinforcement Delivered Date & RN	Learner Objectives Met Date & RN	Not Applicable
D. Antidotes for warfarin			
III. The patient differentiates between common side effects and those warranting a physician's attention.			
IV. The patient discusses other precautions to be taken while on warfarin.			
A. Lists medications to be avoided while taking warfarin.			
B. States who should be contacted in case of injury and describes other emergency measures in case of excessive bleeding.			
C. Describes what precautions are necessary in activities of daily living as a result of taking warfarin.			
D. States how often pro-times must be drawn.			
E. States the importance of wearing a medic alert bracelet at all times.			
V. The patient takes home a booklet on the drug.			

	Content/ Reinforcement Delivered Date & RN	Learner Objectives Met Date & RN	Not Applicable
Evaluation If patient or significant others are unable to complete some or all of this teaching plan, document evaluation in progress notes.			

GUIDELINES: WARFARIN (COUMADIN)

I. The patient explains why warfarin has been prescribed and what effect it has on clotting.

   A. Action of warfarin. *Background for the nurse:* Warfarin reduces coagulation by interfering with prothrombin in its formation of thrombin. It also prevents vitamin K's synthesis of protein in the liver, thus affecting coagulation (increasing the clotting time). The nurse must adapt this information to the patient's level of understanding. The patient needs to know that warfarin prolongs the length of time necessary for blood to clot.

   B. Indications for warfarin use. The drug serves a dual purpose in that it is used both prophylactically and clinically. Prophylactically it is used to prevent a thrombus in patients with a history of thrombophlebitis or phlebitis, vascular disease, mitral valve replacement, recurrent pulmonary emboli, vascular surgery, and any other clotting anomaly or in long-term immobilization of a bedridden patient. Clinically it is used in a patient who has suffered a cerebral vascular accident due to emboli or cerebral emboli to assist in decreasing sludging of blood and in a patient with a current thrombophlebitis.

II. Patient states the following, with regard to the use of warfarin.

   A. Drug dosage. Dosage varies from one patient to another, depending on response to the medication. Dosage is determined by a blood test known as prothrombin time (or PT). The desired PT for a patient on warfarin should be two to two and one-half times that of the control. It is usually documented as

Patient number
Control number

Most patients can maintain an adequate PT on a dosage ranging from 2 to 10 mg of warfarin daily. In rare cases, however, warfarin doses may need to be adjusted above or below this range according to their individual response and PT results. (As mentioned, this drug should be taken daily, preferably with a meal.)

   B. Frequency of administration and what to do if a dose is missed. The patient should be instructed as follows:

     1. Take warfarin at approximately the same time every day. Work with the patient to develop a daily reminder to take warfarin.

     2. Omit a forgotten dose and continue as ordered. If two or more daily doses are missed, contact the physician. The patient should not take an extra dose.

     3. Use a warfarin calendar to facilitate safe administration and refill of the prescription.

   C. The storage of the drug. Keep the drug away from extreme heat or cold (e.g., glove compartment, refrigerator, radiator). This decreases its stability and effectiveness.

   D. The antidote to warfarin. Reassure the patient that there are antidotes that will reverse any severe side effects due to the drug. These are whole blood and vitamin K.

III. The patient differentiates between common side effects and those warranting a physician's attention.

   A. Due to the prolonged bleeding time involved in taking warfarin, a patient must be cautious in all activities. Any excessive bleeding from the nose, gums, ears, and vagina or blood in the urine or stool is abnormal and warrants examination by a physician. Abundance of bruises could indicate further prolonged bleeding time above the desired level, and a PT should be done. A skin rash or lesion also should receive medical attention. Any increased gastrointestinal symptoms, such as excessive diarrhea or vomiting, could alter the vitamin K content in the bowel or cause warfarin loss, since it is excreted in the stool and vomitus. This should be reported to a physician for evaluation.

The drug can be taken with milk to decrease gastrointestinal symptoms. If nausea, vomiting, or diarrhea persist, a physician should be notified.

Advise patients to refill their prescriptions at least a week before their current prescription is empty. A physician should be notified if the prescription has expired or the medication has been misplaced.

   B. If a patient is experiencing a problem with warfarin requiring medical care, the patient is to bring the current pills to the physician so that the dosage can be determined.

IV. The patient discusses other precautions to be taken while on warfarin.

   A. The patient lists medications to be avoided while taking warfarin.

     1. The patient is not to take any medications containing aspirin. Aspirin will increase the bleeding time further and alter the effect of the warfarin. Some common aspirin-containing drugs follow:

Alka-Seltzer	Empirin compound
Allerest	Excedrin
Anacin	Fiorinal
Ascription	Nytol
Bufferin	Percodan
Cough syrups	Some cold remedies
Darvon compound	Vanquish
Dristan	Zacctirin

2. Ascertain that the patient recognizes that many medications can affect the action of warfarin. A physician should be contacted before taking any new medication.

3. The patient is to avoid alcoholic beverages, since they affect clotting time.

B. The patient states who should be contacted about injury and describes other emergency measures in case of excessive bleeding. Patients on warfarin are prone to prolonged bleeding if injured. If any injury should occur, the patient should apply constant pressure until the bleeding stops. If the bleeding continues, a physician should be contacted at once. Be sure that the physician is aware that the patient is taking warfarin.

Have patients alert their dentists about their warfarin prescriptions before any dental work.

C. Describes what precautions are necessary in activities of daily living as a result of taking warfarin. The patient should always use an electric razor when shaving to avoid the possibility of any injury that would result in bleeding.

D. States how often pro-times must be drawn. Most physicians advise a weekly prothrombin time to be done. Arrangements must be made before discharge with either the clinic or family physician. Give the patient some indication of normal results (i.e., 19/10 second, etc.).

E. The patient states the importance of wearing a medic alert bracelet at all times. The patient should always wear a medic alert bracelet or necklace indicating warfarin use. This should be provided by the nurse before discharge.

Part XI

Procedures

	Content/ Reinforcement Delivered Date & RN	Learner Objectives Met Date & RN	Not Applicable

ANGIOGRAPHY

Purpose

To provide the patient with insight into the events before, during, and after angiography procedures.
To help minimize fears or anxieties surrounding the angiography procedure.

Content

   I. Purpose of the diagnostic test, angiography
  II. Pre-angiography events
 III. Events on the day of angiography
 IV. Post-angiography events

Learner Objectives

   I. The patient states the purpose of the test.
     A. Angiography allows the blood vessels of many different areas of the body to be visualized.
     B. By injecting a special dye, any abnormalities (i.e., weakness in vessel wall, sites of internal bleeding, blockages, or abnormal pathways) can be seen on x-ray.
     C. The specific reason for the test is _____.
  II. The patient states the preparations the evening before the test.
     A. A permit is obtained after the procedure is explained.
     B. Pulses above and below the dye injection site may be marked.
     C. Routine chest x-rays, EKGs, and blood tests are completed.
     D. The patient is asked if allergic to dye.
     E. Fluids may be increased according to the physician's orders.
     F. The site of the catheter insertion may be washed and shaved.
     G. A sleeping pill may be offered.
 III. The patient states the events on the day of the procedure.
     A. The diet may vary according to time of test (regular meal, liquids, or NPO).
     B. A hospital gown must be worn; all jewelry will be removed, but rings may be taped on.
     C. The patient is to void before the test.
     D. An oral or intramuscular narcotic is given immediately before leaving the unit to cause drowsiness.

	Content/ Reinforcement Delivered Date & RN	Learner Objectives Met Date & RN	Not Applicable
E. The patient is transported to the procedure room by stretcher and placed on an x-ray table.			
F. Doctors, nurses, and technicians are present. Vital signs are checked and the area is washed and covered with towels.			
G. A needle is inserted to inject the dye via a catheter. X-rays are taken in rapid sequence to follow the dye through the circulation.			

H. The dye injection may cause
  1. Palpitations
  2. Numbness
  3. Flushing
  4. Burning or warm sensation for about 30 seconds			

I. The patient may need to be repositioned at any time during the procedure to aid in the visualization of the desired area.			
J. When completed, the needle catheter is removed, and a thickly padded pressure dressing is applied to the site.			
IV. The patient states the care to be received after the procedure:			

A. Activity
  1. There is strict bedrest from 4 to 12 hours.
  2. The test site limb is kept straight.
  3. A sandbag is placed at the site.			

B. Vital sign monitoring
  1. Blood pressure, heart rate, and respiratory rate are checked frequently.
  2. The dressing site and the pulses above and below the site are checked with each vital sign check.			

C. Hydration 1. Fluids are encouraged per physician's orders.			
Evaluation If patient or significant others are unable to complete some or all of this teaching plan, document evaluation in progress notes.			

	Content/ Reinforcement Delivered Date & RN	Learner Objectives Met Date & RN	Not Applicable

CARDIAC CATHETERIZATION (ADULT)

Purpose

To give information about cardiac catheterization that is easily understood by the patient and family. To lessen patient anxiety about the procedure and elicit cooperation during the catheterization.

Content

   I. Anatomy and physiology of the heart
  II. Atherosclerosis
 III. Angina (refer to angina teaching plan)
 IV. Description of the purpose of cardiac catheterization
  V. Diagnostic tests sometimes done in conjunction with cardiac catheterization
 VI. Description of the cardiac catheterization procedure
VII. Postcatheterization care
VIII. Discharge instructions

Learner Objectives

  I. The patient describes in simple terms the anatomy and physiology of heart muscles including the valves and coronary circulation.
    A. The heart is a hollow muscular organ that pumps blood containing oxygen and nutrients throughout the body.
    B. The valves are located in the heart muscle. They open and close when the heart pumps to protect against the backflow of blood.
    C. The coronary artery system has three major branches. The right coronary artery supplies blood to the right and left side of the heart. The left coronary artery has two branches and carries blood to the left side of the heart.

 II. The patient describes atherosclerosis.
    A. Fatty layers (plaques) form and accumulate on the lining of the blood vessels that feed the heart muscle (coronary arteries).
    B. Fatty substances are made of cholesterol.
    C. These fatty substances clog the blood vessels and cause a decrease in the amount of blood that gets to the heart muscle.

III. The patient describes the physiology of angina by completing the angina teaching plan, if needed.

	Content/ Reinforcement Delivered Date & RN	Learner Objectives Met Date & RN	Not Applicable
IV. The patient describes the purpose of a cardiac catheterization.			
A. Cardiac catheterization is a procedure that assists in an examination of the heart.			
B. Using a catheter, injected dye, and x-rays, the valves, chambers, and blood vessels supplying the heart are visualized.			
C. This permits diagnosis of problems involving the heart.			
V. The patient describes the tests done before and after cardiac catheterization and discusses in general terms why they are done:			
A. EKG. This test shows the heart rate and rhythm. It may also show evidence of heart injury.			
B. Ultrasound or echocardiogram. This test uses high-frequency sound waves to visualize the heart in motion and shows the size of the heart. It can also identify malfunctioning heart valves.			
C. Cardiac series. Indicates the size of the heart chambers and action of the heart at work. The patient drinks a small amount of barium, and an x-ray is taken.			
D. Lipid profile. Blood tests to measure the fats in the blood.			
E. Stress test. Usually performed on a stationary bicycle or treadmill under the supervision of a physician. It helps determine how much activity can be performed. It also assists in making a diagnosis of coronary artery disease.			
F. Thallium stress test. The same as a regular stress test but with the use of a radioactive isotope, which is injected into the arm to visualize the blood supply to the heart muscle.			
VI. The patient describes in simple terms the cardiac catheterization procedure:			
A. Skin preparation			
1. The hair is shaved and the skin washed with an antibacterial soap.			
2. The sites for skin preparation are inside the right elbow and right underarm and the right and left groins.			
B. Catheterization procedure			
1. The patient is placed on the table with an overhead x-ray tube and camera.			
2. An EKG machine is attached and continuously monitors the heartbeat.			
3. The skin is again washed with antibacterial soap and covered with sterile towels and drapes.			
4. The arm and groin sites are anesthetized.			

	Content/ Reinforcement Delivered Date & RN	Learner Objectives Met Date & RN	Not Applicable
5. The right heart catheterization is done via the right arm and groin veins. A small incision is made into the right arm vein. A catheter is moved through the vein to the right side of the heart where blood samples and pressure measurements are taken.			
6. The left heart catheterization uses the large artery in the groin or the artery in the arm. A catheter is advanced through the artery to the left side of the heart where pressure measurements are taken. An x-ray camera is used to take pictures of the heart's function.			
7. Dye is injected at various times during the catheterization to permit visualization of the heart via x-ray. When the dye is injected, the patient may feel sensations of warmth, develop a rash, or have feelings of nausea or headache. Although these sensations are common, they should be reported to the doctor or nurse when experienced.			

8. At the end of the procedures,
   a) All catheters are removed.
   b) The right arm incision is sutured.
   c) Hand pressure is applied to the groin area for 15 to 20 minutes to stop any bleeding.
   d) Pressure dressings are applied to each area.			

VII. The patient states in simple terms the postcatheterization care:			
A. First 24 hours			
1. Vital signs will be checked frequently when the patient returns to the floor. Wrist and foot pulses and other vital signs are monitored.			
2. Pressure dressings on the right arm and groin will be observed when vital signs are taken.			

3. If the groin site is used,
    a) A sandbag will be placed over the pressure dressing for 8 to 10 hours.
    b) The leg must be straight and bedrest maintained for 12 to 24 hours.
    c) The head of the bed will be raised slightly.
    d) A urinal and/or bedpan will be available and the nurse will assist with their use.			

4. Fluids will be given per doctor's orders.			
5. Pain medication will be ordered. The patient should ask the nurse for medication as needed for pain or discomfort.			
B. Day-after procedure			
1. Pressure dressings are changed or removed.			
2. The sutures in the right arm are covered with gauze dressing.			

	Content/ Reinforcement Delivered Date & RN	Learner Objectives Met Date & RN	Not Applicable

3. Catheterization results are discussed with the doctor.
VIII. Patient states discharge instructions:
    A. Reason to contact the physician
      1. Fever
      2. Drainage from catheterization sites (arm or groin)
      3. Bruising at arm or groin
      4. Increased pain in catheterization sites
    B. Follow-up
      1. Next appointment: _____
      2. Physician #: _____
         Emergency room #: _____
Patient or significant others have met objectives of other related teaching plans:
   Angina teaching plan
   Congestive heart failure teaching plan
   Hypertension teaching plan			

Evaluation If patient or significant others are unable to complete some or all of this teaching plan, document evaluation in progress notes.			

	Content/ Reinforcement Delivered Date & RN	Learner Objectives Met Date & RN	Not Applicable

LUMBAR PUNCTURE

Purpose

To ensure the patient's understanding of a lumbar puncture and compliance with the preparation and procedure.

Content

I. Explanation of the purpose of the lumbar puncture as it applies to the patient
II. Description of the preprocedure preparations
III. Description of the lumbar puncture procedure
IV. Explanation of postprocedure care

Learner Objectives

I. The patient states that the lumbar puncture is a procedure that collects cerebrospinal fluid for evaluation and measures the pressure in the cerebrospinal system. It is used to help diagnose the patient's condition so that treatment can be initiated or evaluated.

II. The patient describes and demonstrates preparation for the procedure:
   A. The patient will be asked to void before the lumbar puncture.
   B. The patient assumes a side-lying position in bed with the head flexed so that the chin is on the chest. The knees are drawn up toward the abdomen. The physician performing the procedure is behind the patient.

III. The patient describes the lumbar puncture procedure.
   A. The physician administers a local anesthetic to the back in the area where the procedure will be performed.
   B. As the needle is inserted in the lumbar spinal space, a slight pressure will be felt.
   C. The physician first measures the opening pressure and then collects specimens of spinal fluid for testing.
   D. When the procedure is finished, the physician removes the needle and applies a Band-Aid to the site.

IV. The patient describes postprocedure care. The patient will be asked to:
   A. Remain flat for 8 hours.
   B. Drink liquids to prevent dehydration.
   C. Alert nurses to the need for pain medication for headache.

	Content/ Reinforcement Delivered Date & RN	Learner Objectives Met Date & RN	Not Applicable
Evaluation If patient or significant others are unable to complete some or all of the teaching plan, document evaluation in progress notes.			

	Content/ Reinforcement Delivered Date & RN	Learner Objectives Met Date & RN	Not Applicable

ORAL CHOLECYSTOGRAPHY

Purpose

To instruct and prepare the patient for x-rays of the gallbladder.

Content

  I. The gallbladder and its function
 II. Description of the x-ray examination
III. Dietary preparation for the procedure
IV. Handout

Learner Objectives

  I. The patient describes the gallbladder.
    A. The patient locates the gallbladder on own body (upper right quadrant of body).
    B. The patient states that the gallbladder assists in the digestion of food.
    C. The patient describes symptoms that warrant a cholecystography: nausea, vomiting, pain, intolerance for fatty foods.
 II. The patient describes the oral cholecystography procedure.
    A. The patient states that the evening before the exam radiopaque dye tablets known as _____ are taken per the doctor's order.
    B. The patient states that the x-ray tests the gallbladder's ability to store dye. This helps to determine how well the gallbladder functions.
    C. The patient describes the examination as painless.
    D. The patient states that the examination takes 30 to 45 minutes. If the examination is done on an outpatient basis, extra time must be allowed to determine that the x-ray films have developed properly.
III. The patient states that eating and drinking are not permitted from midnight before the exam until the exam is finished.
IV. If the test performed on outpatient basis, an instruction handout is taken home.

Evaluation

If patient or significant others are unable to complete some or all of this teaching plan, document evaluation in progress notes.

GUIDELINES: ORAL CHOLECYSTOGRAPHY

I. The patient locates the gallbladder on own body and describes its function.

    The gallbladder is located in the right upper quadrant of the abdomen. It stores and secretes bile, which is used in the digestion of foods. The components of bile can cause the formation of stones that obstruct bile passages. Symptoms of gallbladder dysfunction may include acute onset of nausea, vomiting, and pain. Food intolerance may also be noted with fried or fatty foods. A diagnostic gallbladder series is ordered if gallbladder dysfunction is suspected.

II. The patient verbally describes the procedure. The oral gallbladder series (cholecystography) is the most common type of diagnostic x-ray taken for studying gallbladder function. The evening before the examination radiopaque dye tablets are taken by the patient as prescribed. The patient should take the tablets at 5-minute intervals to prevent nausea and to prevent the gallbladder from expelling the dye because of rapid digestion. The x-ray measures the gallbladder's ability to store the dye, which reflects gallbladder function. The following morning the patient goes to the x-ray suite. (A wheelchair or stretcher is used if the patient is hospitalized.) X-rays are taken and because they cannot penetrate the dye, a shadow of the gallbladder should appear. Because gallstones are not radiopaque, they show up as dark areas on the x-ray. Once the x-rays are completed, the patient may return to the hospital floor or home. A regular or prescribed diet may be resumed. There is no special care after the examination. The total time for the examination is 30 to 45 minutes. Most of the patient's time is spent in waiting for x-ray results. If the x-ray study is done on an outpatient basis, the patient should plan to be involved with the procedure most of the morning.

III. The patient describes dietary restrictions necessary for the x-ray examination.

    The day before the exam there are no special restrictions. The patient, however, must take nothing by mouth after midnight the night before the exam and fast until after the exam has taken place.

IV. Handout

    If the test is done on an outpatient basis, an instruction handout is given to the patient and reviewed.

	Content/ Reinforcement Delivered	Learner Objectives Met	Not Applicable
	Date & RN	Date & RN	

METRIZAMIDE MYELOGRAM

Purpose

To familiarize the patient and family with all aspects of the myelogram in order to diminish anxiety and to promote maximum patient participation during and after the procedure.

Content

    I. Purpose of the procedure
   II. Description of the procedure
  III. Description of routine care for before and after the myelogram
  IV. Review of the reasons to contact the physician after discharge
   V. Follow-up instructions

Learner Objectives

    I. The patient describes in general terms the purpose of a myelogram.
      A. It is a diagnostic test used to visualize the spinal cord.
      B. Some of the abnormalities that can be identified with this test are protruding discs, tumors, cysts, and other lesions.
      C. The patient states: "The reason for my myelogram is _____."

   II. The patient describes the procedure in general terms.
      A. It is performed in the radiology department by a physician.
      B. The physician anesthetizes the lower back in the area of the procedure.
      C. The patient assumes a side lying position with the knees bent toward the chest. This position increases the space between the vertebrae of the spine.
      D. A needle is inserted into the lumbar spinal space and a slight pressure is felt.
      E. A small amount of spinal fluid that is present in the spinal column is removed.
      F. A liquid contrast dye is injected, and the table is tilted in various positions to allow the dye to outline the area surrounding the spinal cord.
      G. X-rays are taken.
      H. After the x-rays, the patient is returned to the unit. The dye is not removed. It will be absorbed by the body and excreted in the urine over the following 24 to 48 hours.

	Content/ Reinforcement Delivered	Learner Objectives Met	Not Applicable
	Date & RN	Date & RN	

III. The patient describes in general terms the routine to be followed before and after the myelogram:
A. Preparation
  1. Solid food is withheld on the day of the procedure.
  2. Clear liquids are allowed and a liberal intake is encouraged to assure proper hydration.
B. Vital signs
  1. Vital signs are taken frequently after the procedure.
  2. Pulse rate, temperature, and blood pressure are taken at least every 4 hours following the test.
  3. Neurological status is checked with vital signs. The nurse will ask the patient to move all extremities. The nurse should be notified if the patient experiences changes in sensation or movement, neck pain, headache, or nausea.
  4. Pain medication is available for discomfort. The nurse is to be informed if discomfort occurs and is not relieved by the medication.
C. Positioning
  1. The patient is restricted to bedrest for 24 hours after the procedure.
  2. Immediately following the procedure the head is elevated at least 30°. This is done to decrease the chance of common side effects such as headache and nausea.
  3. The patient's head will be elevated for 8 hours, then the patient will lie flat in bed for 24 hours.
D. Hydration
  1. The patient should drink at least 3 quarts of fluid during the first 24 hours following the procedure unless medically contraindicated.
  2. The amount of fluids consumed and the amount of urine passed are measured by the nurse.
  3. Hydration is important as it helps the body to excrete the dye.
E. Bedpan and/or urinal use
  1. It is necessary to use a bedpan and/or urinal while the patient is on bedrest. This should be practiced before the procedure.
IV. The patient states the reasons to contact the physician after discharge:
A. The patient should report:
  1. Any changes in the color of the feet or hands
  2. Any numbness or tingling
  3. Decreased movement of any extremity
  4. Stiff neck
  5. Severe headache
  6. Fever			

	Content/ Reinforcement Delivered Date & RN	Learner Objectives Met Date & RN	Not Applicable
V. The patient states the date and time of the follow-up appointment and important phone numbers: Follow-up appointment: _____ Physician #: _____ Emergency room #: _____ Orthopedic clinic #: _____			

Evaluation

If patient or significant others are unable to complete some or all of this teaching plan, document evaluation in progress notes.

	Content/ Reinforcement Delivered Date & RN	Learner Objectives Met Date & RN	Not Applicable

UPPER GASTROINTESTINAL SERIES
 	
Purpose
 	
To provide the patient with information explaining the procedure and its use as a diagnostic test.
 	
Content
 	
   I. Purpose of an upper gastrointestinal series (UGI)
     A. Anatomy and physiology
     B. Clinical indications
  II. Preparation
 III. Procedure
 IV. Postprocedure care
  V. Handout			

Learner Objectives
 	
   I. The patient describes an UGI.
     A. An UGI is a special x-ray examination (fluoroscopy) of the esophagus and stomach. It is sometimes combined with a small bowel follow-through, which allows examination of the small intestines. The x-rays are performed after the patient drinks a radiopaque substance called *barium*.
     B. The patient explains why the examination has been ordered.
  II. The patient describes the preparation for the examination.
     A. The patient is asked to increase fluid intake the day before the examination.
     B. The patient states that eating and drinking are prohibited from midnight before the examination.
 III. The patient describes the sequence of events and sensations felt during the procedure.
     A. The patient is placed on a special table that rotates in horizontal, vertical, and semivertical positions. A physician or technician assists the patient in turning on the stomach, back, and side.
     B. The patient drinks a thick, chalky, flavored, milk-shake-type drink (barium).
     C. A series of x-rays is taken as barium passes through the gastrointestinal tract and outlines the contours.
     D. If a small bowel follow-through is done, the examination takes longer. The passage of barium is followed as it leaves the stomach and enters the intestines. A series of pictures is taken.			

	Content/Reinforcement Delivered Date & RN	Learner Objectives Met Date & RN	Not Applicable

E. The patient may feel pressure or discomfort if the abdomen is palpated or compressed to allow adequate coating of the intestinal and stomach lining.
F. The patient may feel nauseated, bloated, or have indigestion after drinking barium.
IV. The patient defines post-UGI care.
  A. A laxative may be given to encourage passage of barium.
  B. Adequate fluid intake is encouraged.
  C. The stool will be light (chalky) in color for 24 to 72 hours as the barium is excreted.
  D. Other abdominal or kidney x-rays cannot be visualized adequately until the barium passes through the system.
  E. Preliminary results are available the day of the tests; final results are reported several days later.
V. The patient takes a handout home.			

Evaluation

If patient or significant others are unable to complete some or all of this teaching plan, document evaluation in progress notes.

Part XII

Miscellaneous

	Content/ Reinforcement Delivered	Learner Objectives Met	Not Applicable
	Date & RN	Date & RN	

GENERAL DISCHARGE

Purpose

To prepare the patient for discharge from the hospital or transfer to another facility.

Content

   I. Explanation of what caused hospitalization and what has been done to treat the problem

  II. Discussion of what, if any, residual effects of a condition or procedure may be expected

 III. Review of posthospital home care

    A. Teaching and demonstration of any procedures that may have to be done at home

    B. Teaching of other necessary measures utilizing proper guides and handouts

    C. Review specific teaching plans related to illness

 IV. Explanation of provision for follow-up care

  V. Explanation of what the patient may expect if posthospital plan includes transfer to another facility

Learner Objectives

   I. The patient states in simple terms the diagnosis and what was done to treat the problem in the hospital.

_____

_____

  II. The patient states what, if any, normal residual effects of the condition and subsequent procedures may be expected.

_____

_____

 III. The patient reviews home care.

    A. The patient explains and demonstrates procedures that may have to be done at home and, if necessary, how to obtain and maintain equipment or supplies.

_____

_____

    B. The patient explains other treatments prescribed and demonstrates knowledge of these measures, i.e., medications, diet.

_____

_____

	Content/ Reinforcement Delivered Date & RN	Learner Objectives Met Date & RN	Not Applicable

C. The patient meets objectives of the following teaching plans related to illness.
 	
_____
_____
 	
IV. The patient states follow-up instructions:
    A. Reasons to call physician:
        1. _____
        2. _____
        3. _____
        4. _____
        5. _____
    B. Numbers to call if problems:
        1. Physician #: _____
        2. Emergency room #: _____
        3. _____
    C. The patient states that a follow-up appointment is scheduled on _____ with _____.
    D. The patient states the community agencies that will be used, how to make contact, what services are provided, and how payment will be made.
 	
_____
_____
 	
V. If applicable, the patient states the name and address of the next facility, how long a stay is anticipated, the reason for transfer, general description of facility, and how payment will be made.
 	
_____
_____			

Evaluation If patient or significant others are unable to complete some or all of this teaching plan, document evaluation in progress notes.			

	Content/ Reinforcement Delivered Date & RN	Learner Objectives Met Date & RN	Not Applicable

FEVER IN CHILDREN

Purpose

To teach parents or guardians how to care for their child with a fever at home.

Content

    I. Definition of normal temperature and fever
   II. Management of temperature elevation
      A. Importance of a thermometer in the home
      B. Demonstration of how to take a temperature
      C. Demonstration of how to read the thermometer
      D. Demonstration of thermometer care
  III. How to administer antipyretics, including name, dosage, and frequency
  IV. Other fever control measures
      A. Light clothing
      B. Adequate fluids
      C. Bathing
      D. Room temperature
   V. Indications for notifying a physician
  VI. How to contact the physician

Learner Objectives

    I. The parent states that a normal temperature is 37°C or 98.6°F. The parent or patient defines fever as a temperature elevated higher than 38°C or 101°F.
   II. The parent discusses management of an elevated temperature.
      A. States that a thermometer is available at home or describes how to obtain one.
      B. The parent demonstrates and describes how to take a temperature.
         1. Takes thermometer out of container and rinses with cool water.
         2. Shakes the thermometer until the mercury line is below the numbers.
         3. Stays with the child during the procedure.
           a) *Oral*
             (1) Puts the bulb end of the oral thermometer under the patient's tongue for 5 to 8 minutes.
             (2) Asks the child to keep the mouth and lips closed but not to bite the thermometer.

	Content/ Reinforcement Delivered Date & RN	Learner Objectives Met Date & RN	Not Applicable

(3) After 5 to 8 minutes, takes the thermometer out, holds up to eye level, and reads.
b) *Rectal*
  (1) Puts a small amount of lubricating jelly on a tissue or cotton ball.
  (2) Lubricates the bulb of the rectal thermometer. The rectal thermometer bulb is smaller and wider than an oral thermometer.
  (3) Lays a child on the back, side, or abdomen.
  (4) Inserts the thermometer 1 inch through the anus into the rectum and holds in place for 3 minutes.
  (5) Takes out and wipes off the thermometer, holding it up to eye level to read.
c) *Axillary*
  (1) Dries the child's axilla (armpit).
  (2) Places the bulb of an oral thermometer in the center of the armpit, the axilla.
  (3) The thermometer should be held upright by placing the child's arm across the chest or at the side, with the arm snug against the body.
  (4) Stays with the child.
  (5) Leaves the thermometer in place for 10 minutes.
  (6) Removes and holds up to eye level to read.
C. The parent demonstrates how to read the thermometer.
  1. Holds the thermometer at eye level by the end opposite the bulb.
  2. Withdraws and rotates the thermometer until the column of mercury and the row of numbers can be seen.
  3. Identifies correctly the patient's temperature.
D. The parent demonstrates how to care for a thermometer.
  1. After using the thermometer, cleans it in warm (not hot) soapy water, rinses thoroughly with cool water, and dries it.
  2. Stores the thermometer in a container to prevent breakage.
E. The parent states that the temperature should be taken every four (4) hours until it is below 38.5°C or 100°F.
 	
III. The parent meets the objectives of the medication teaching plan for the antipyretic prescribed and identifies the name, dose, frequency, and time to administer.
 	
A. The parents take an antipyretic handout home.			

	Content/ Reinforcement Delivered Date & RN	Learner Objectives Met Date & RN	Not Applicable

IV. The parent describes the appropriate action to be taken in addition to antipyretics.
  A. Dress the child in light clothing.
  B. Feed the child adequate fluids. Increase fluids to prevent or correct dehydration.
    The child should have _____cc/24 hours
  C. If the temperature is not controlled by these actions and antipyretics, the child can be made comfortable by immersion in a tub of lukewarm (not cold) water for 15 to 20 minutes.
  D. Keep the room temperature comfortably cool.
V. The parent describes indications for notifying a physician:
  A. Persistent fever
  B. Occurrence of rash, irritability, lethargy, poor feeding, sleeplessness, vomiting, diarrhea, complaint of pain or discomfort
  C. The occurrence of dehydration as manifested by dry lips and oral mucosa, decreased urine output, absence of tears, and poor skin turgor
  D. Febrile seizure
VI. The parent states the date of the return visit or telephone number to call if problems or questions arise:
  Date: _____
  Telephone: _____			

Evaluation If patient or significant others are unable to complete some or all of this teaching plan, document evaluation in progress notes.			

	Content/ Reinforcement Delivered Date & RN	Learner Objectives Met Date & RN	Not Applicable
INTRODUCTION TO INTENSIVE CARE UNIT **Purpose** To reduce the anxiety of the patient and a significant other by an introduction to the intensive care unit and the staff of the unit. To promote cooperation during the intensive care stay. **Content** I. Discussion of the reason for the ICU admission and the expected length of stay II. Explanation of the role of the ICU nurse III. Explanation of the role of the physicians (attending physicians, residents, interns) and the role of medical students and physician assistants when available IV. Explanation of the roles of members of support service departments V. Discussion of the policies of the unit VI. Explanation of the physical and sensory aspects of the intensive care setting VII. Pamphlet reviewed if available **Learner Objectives** I. The patient and significant other state the reason for admission and the expected length of stay.			

II. The patient and significant other describe the role of the ICU nurse.
III. The patient and significant other describe the roles of the physicians, medical students, physician assistants.
IV. The patient and significant other describe the roles of support service department members such as respiratory therapy, chest physical therapy, x-ray technician.
V. The patient and significant other describe unit policies.
  A. Permission to enter the unit is obtained via
    1. Telephone _____
    2. Doorbell _____
  B. The call-in policy. One family member is to be appointed a spokesperson.
    Name of spokesperson _____			

	Content/ Reinforcement Delivered Date & RN	Learner Objectives Met Date & RN	Not Applicable
C. The number of visitors is limited to two at one time			
D. Visiting may be limited so that the medical care of the patient is not interrupted or jeopardized			
E. Visiting may be denied for procedures or the patient's need for rest			
VI. The patient and significant other describe the physical and sensory aspects inherent in the intensive care setting:			
A. Physical			
1. Alarms—usually interference			
2. Intravenous lines—necessary to have access to a vein at all times			
3. Respirators—inability to talk, frequent suctioning			
4. Vital signs—frequency			
5. Various testing—electrocardiograms, chest x-rays, blood drawing			
6. Drains—nasogastric tube, chest tubes, Foley catheter			
7. Weighing—usually every day			
8. Use of commode and urinal			
9. Use of a footboard			
10. Deep breathing exercises			
11. Activity level progression			
12. Diet—variable			
B. Sensory			
1. Noise level			
2. Lack of sleep			
3. Perceptual disturbances; concept of time, place, and person			
4. Bedrest			
VII. The patient and the family read and take home the ICU pamphlet, if available.			

Evaluation

If patient or significant others are unable to complete some or all of this teaching plan, document evaluation in progress notes.

	Content/ Reinforcement Delivered Date & RN	Learner Objectives Met Date & RN	Not Applicable

INTRODUCTION TO PRIMARY NURSING
 	
Purpose
 	
To foster the patient's and family's understanding of the function of a primary nurse.
 	
Content
 	
    I. Definition of a primary nurse
   II. Expectations of a primary nurse
  III. Identification of the primary nurse
  IV. Description of where the name of the patient's primary nurse can be found
   V. Explanation of the assessment, goals, and care plan
  VI. Review of resource people
 	
Learner Objectives			

I. The patient and family define what a primary nurse is.
     A. The primary nurse is the nurse who is responsible for overseeing the nursing care that the patient (and family members) will receive during the hospitalization.
   II. The patient and family describe what they can expect of a primary nurse.
     A. The primary nurse will discuss nursing care and special needs with the patient.
     B. Together the primary nurse and patient will plan how the patient's needs will be met.
     C. The primary nurse will work closely with the patient's doctors and other hospital personnel to coordinate nursing care.
     D. The primary nurse will teach the patient and family about health needs, e.g., medication and diet teaching.
     E. The primary nurse will keep the patient and family informed about health progress.
     F. The patient indicates the necessity to communicate needs, concerns, fears, and expectations to the primary nurse.
  III. The patient and family identify the primary nurse by full name and describe coverage when the primary nurse is off duty.
     A. The patient states the primary nurse's full name.			

	Content/ Reinforcement Delivered	Learner Objectives Met	Not Applicable
	Date & RN	Date & RN	

B. The primary nurse will notify the patient when scheduled to be off and who will be following the case during this time.

IV. The patient and family state where they can find the name of the primary nurse:
  A. Primary nursing board. A board at the nursing station where the patient and family can find their primary nurse's name.
  B. _____
  _____.
  C. _____
  _____.

V. The patient and family describe in simple terms the nursing assessment, care plan, and patient goals:
  A. Nursing assessment. Helps identify the patient's health needs that should be addressed.
  B. Care plan. A list of problems and goals that the primary nurse and patient have identified and will focus on during this hospitalization.
  C. Goals. The patient and family identify at least one problem and goal that the primary nurse and patient have as a focus.
  Problem

  _____
  _____.

  Goal

  _____
  _____.

VI. The patient and family state resources that they may use to answer questions.
  A. Patient and family state that they will keep a list of questions.
  B. Patient and family state resources including
    1. Primary nurse
    2. Physicians, residents, interns, medical students
    3. Specialty nurses, therapists, technicians
      a. Ostomy nurse
      b. Physical therapist
      c. Occupational therapist
      d. Dietitian

Evaluation

If patient or significant others are unable to complete some or all of this teaching plan, document evaluation in progress notes.

	Content/ Reinforcement Delivered	Learner Objectives Met	Not Applicable
	Date & RN	Date & RN	

GENERAL PREOPERATIVE PATIENT

Purpose

To explain the routine preoperative and postoperative procedures. To lessen the patient's preoperative anxiety and to promote patient cooperation during the postoperative phase.

Content

    I. Operative procedure
   II. Preoperative tests and laboratory work
 III. Routine events before surgery in the patient care area
 IV. Routine events before surgery in the operating room holding area
   V. Operating room environment
 VI. Routine events after surgery

Learner Objectives

    I. The patient describes the operating procedure.
       A. Name _____
       B. Length of procedure _____
       C. Reasons for procedure

         _____

       D. Anatomy and physiology involved

         _____

   II. The patient describes in general terms preoperative tests and laboratory work.
       A. Blood and urine samples are done to help evaluate preoperative health status.
       B. Electrocardiogram is done to evaluate cardiac status.
       C. Chest x-rays assess respiratory status.
 III. The patient describes in general terms the routine events before surgery in the patient care area.
       A. To decrease lung irritation and secretions, smoking is discouraged.
       B. The skin around the operative area may be shaved and washed to reduce the bacteria on the skin (if applicable).
       C. An enema may be given to prevent complications during surgery and promote comfort after surgery.
       D. After an explanation of the procedure, the physician requests that the patient sign permission for surgery.

	Content/ Reinforcement Delivered Date & RN	Learner Objectives Met Date & RN	Not Applicable
E. Medication given by intramuscular injection induces relaxation and drowsiness.			
F. Nothing by mouth is permitted after midnight the night before surgery to empty the gastrointestinal tract and reduce nausea and vomiting.			
G. Transportation to the operating room is by stretcher.			
IV. The patient describes routine events in the operating room holding area.			
A. If the skin is not shaved and washed in the patient's room, it may be done in the holding area.			
B. Intravenous solution is started, usually in the arm, to provide fluids and administer medication.			
C. EKG pads and blood pressure cuffs are attached to monitor cardiac status.			
D. There is a family waiting area on the same floor as the operating room where families can stay during surgery.			
V. The patient describes in general terms the operating room environment.			
A. The operating table is firm and narrow.			
B. The temperature of the room is cool, but blankets are available to keep the patient warm. The patient should let the nurse know if a blanket is needed.			
C. The doctors and nurses are dressed in hats and masks.			
VI. The patient describes in general terms the routine postoperative events.			
A. The patient remains in the recovery room until awake and vital signs are stable.			
B. The surgical incision is covered with a dressing.			
C. The patient is asked to turn, cough, and deep breathe every 15 minutes to help move secretions out of the lungs.			
D. An intravenous line usually remains in place to administer fluids and medication.			
E. A cardiac monitor is attached to evaluate cardiac status.			
F. A nurse takes vital signs every 15 minutes immediately after surgery to monitor response to treatment. The frequency will diminish as the patient becomes stable after surgery.			
G. The family may visit after the patient has returned to the unit.			
H. Ambulation is usually allowed the evening after surgery depending on the patient's condition.			
I. Pain medication will be ordered and the patient should tell the nurse when it is needed.			

	Content/ Reinforcement Delivered	Learner Objectives Met	Not Applicable
	Date & RN	Date & RN	
Evaluation If patient or significant others are unable to complete some or all of this teaching plan, document evaluation in progress notes.			

GUIDELINES: GENERAL ADULT PREOPERATIVE

II. The patient describes the basic preoperative tests and laboratory work. Blood and urine specimens help the physician assess a patient's general overall health before surgery. The patient also has an electrocardiogram (EKG). This is done by placing leads (metal squares) on the patient and acquiring an electrical representation of heart function. This electrical representation is seen on a strip of graph paper, which comes out of the EKG machine. From this information the doctor can assess the patient's cardiac status.

On the day before surgery, the patient may also have a chest x-ray. This is done to help the physician assess the patient's respiratory health. Because anesthesia causes increased buildup of secretions, it is important to note the health status of the lungs before surgery.

III. The patient describes the routine before surgery in the patient care area.

A. No cigarette smoking. The patient is asked not to smoke if possible or to reduce the amount of smoking as much as possible. During the administration of anesthesia, secretions tend to build up in the lungs. If a patient smokes, smoke causes irritation in the lungs and the lungs build up even more secretions. Lung congestion can contribute to the postoperative development of pneumonia.

B. Skin preparation. On the evening before surgery, the patient's skin may be prepared for surgery. The skin around the incisional area is shaved and washed. This is done because hair harbors bacteria that could cause wound infection. This procedure may also be done just before surgery in the preoperative area.

C. Enema. To prevent complications during and comfort after surgery, the doctor may order an enema given the evening before surgery.

D. Operative permit. The patient needs to sign a permit (consent form) before surgery. Explain to the patient that this is done to document that the patient consented to the surgery and understood fully the nature of the procedure. Encourage the patient to ask questions before signing the permit.

E. Medications. The patient is offered a sleeping pill the night before surgery. Depending on the type of surgery to be performed, the patient may receive preoperative antibiotics. This is done to increase resistance to infection during the postoperative period. When the patient is called to go to the OR (operating room), medications by

intramuscular injection are given to induce relaxation and drowsiness. Explain to the patient that the siderails will be raised in order to ensure safety. This is done for all patients who have received preoperative medication.

F. Nothing by mouth (NPO) after midnight. Explain to the patient that NPO means nothing by mouth. During surgery it is important to have an empty gastrointestinal tract to prevent nausea and vomiting, which may be caused by the anesthesia.

G. Transportation to the operating room. The patient is transported to the operating room on a stretcher.

Explain to the patients that a hospital gown will be worn; their wedding bands will be secured by tape. They cannot wear any other articles of jewelry to the operating room because of possible loss.

IV. The patient describes in general terms the routine events in the operating room holding area. The patient arrives by stretcher to an anesthesia or holding area. This is an area outside the operating room where an intravenous infusion of fluid is started. It is called an IV. People may be wearing masks. It is important for the patient to know that even if the attendants are wearing masks, they can still talk. The patient should feel free to ask questions.

V. The patient describes the daily routine after surgery.

A. Recovery room. After the surgical procedure is completed, the patient goes to the recovery room. Let the patient know that there are other patients in the recovery room, and not to be alarmed by seeing and hearing other patients. Vital signs, blood pressure, and temperature are monitored frequently by a nurse in the recovery room. Explain to the patient that this is normal procedure and that the frequency will diminish as recovery from anesthesia proceeds. One of the recovery room nurses accompanies the patient back to the unit.

B. Surgical dressing. The patient should expect to have bandages over the incisional area. The nurse will be checking the dressing frequently to make sure that there is no bleeding or excess drainage.

C. Respiratory treatment

1. Turning, deep breathing, and coughing. On returning to the room, the patient will be asked to turn, deep breathe, and cough at least every 2 hours. During surgery, secretions accumulate in the lungs. It is important that these secretions be coughed up because a buildup of secretions in the lungs may cause

pneumonia and fever. The nurse should illustrate deep breathing and coughing.

2. The patient may also have IPPB (intermittent positive pressure breathing) treatment ordered. This treatment is designed to help inflate the lungs, so that secretions might be loosened. It is done by a machine that is connected to compressed air. As the patient takes a breath, air is forced into the lungs, causing them to expand. After the treatment, the patient is encouraged to cough.

3. A blow glove is another device that helps the patient take deeper breaths. A plastic glove is attached to the barrel of a 50-cc irrigation syringe. The patient is asked to blow into the glove as if it were a balloon. This forces the patient to take deep breaths. The incentive spirometer and Triflo blow balls may also be used to achieve similar results.

D. Intravenous lines. After surgery, the patient may continue to have an intravenous solution infusion. The reason for continuing such a solution is to provide fluids and a means to give medications. Also, during surgery, the patient loses body fluids and blood through the incision. It is therefore essential that these fluids are replaced.

E. Cardiac monitor. A cardiac monitor continues to be attached in the recovery room. This allows the nurses and physicians to evaluate the patient's cardiac status. The monitor may be removed before the patient returns to the floor, but the patient may continue to be monitored while on the floor.

F. Family visitation. The patient's family is kept informed about the progress of surgery. Visiting hours begin at _____ so that they may be able to visit soon after the patient returns to the room. Exceptions can be made to allow a family member to see the patient before official visiting hours.

G. Ambulation. Usually the patient is allowed out of bed the day after the surgery. Give the patient an idea of how long bedrest will be necessary for the specific type of surgery and document this. By walking soon after surgery, the patient is better able to bring up secretions in the lungs. Remind the patient that after surgery it is normal to feel weak, so during the first walk the nurse should be asked for assistance.

H. Medications. Pain medication is ordered and the patient should not hesitate to ask for it. It is normal to have discomfort after surgery. The medication is usually prescribed to be given intramuscularly every 3 to 4 hours. The patient should let the nurse know if the medication relieved the discomfort. Remind the patient that it is better to ask for the medication before the pain becomes severe.

Evaluation and Follow-up

Generally evaluate how the patient received your teaching. Was the person an eager learner or too anxious to absorb the teaching? Indicate if you have recommendations for further reinforcement of teaching.

Note: Some ideas were gained from Brunner's *Textbook of Medical Surgical Nursing.*

CONTRIBUTORS

Deborah Canty-Goodie, RN, BSN
Margaret Davoren, RN, BSN
Kathleen Bower, RN, MSN
Joyce Caron, RN
Jean McCorry, RN, BS
Mary Gutowski, RN
Janet Troski, RN
Joni Beshansky, RN
Susan Goldberg, RN, BSN
Celeste Cuddemi, RN, BSN
Joan Kraus, RN, BSN
Denise Richards, RN, BSN
Cathy Noble, RN, BSN
Karen Esckilsen, RN, BSN
Kathleen Adams, RN, BSN, MSN
Denise Paone, RN, BSN
Cindi Galligan, RN, BSN
Donna Euerle, RN, MSN
Sally Johnson, RN, MSN
Laurie Luke, RN, BSN
Cheryl Roffo, RN
Coleen Kirk, RN, BSN
Nancy Lyga, RN, BSN, MSN
Cynthia Strong, RN
Linda Donovan, RN, BSN
Paula Bray, RN, BSN
Nancy Mansueto, RN, BSN, MSN
Judith Clevesy Carleo, RN, BSN
Marge Bedard, RN, AD
Lisa Novicki, RN
Ginny Ryan-Morrell, RN
Ellen Howard, RN
Barbara MacLean, RN, BS
Patricia McLaughlin, RN, BSN
Shelley MacDonald, RN, BSN
Susan Dunn, RN
Michelle McIntosh, RN, MSN
Eileen Crawfort, RN, BA
Donna Melanson, RN
Kathleen Scully, RN, BSN
Mary Wenners, RN, AD
Shirley Chimi, RN
Rita McCarthy, RN, BSN, MSN
Clroia Clear, RN
Patricia Bruno, RN, BSN
Nancy Gilman, RN
Charla Scott, RN, BSN

Carol Reilly, RN, BSN
Jacki Frost, RN
Ellen Gaffney, RN, BSN
Amy Murdoch, RN, BSN
Mary Cooney, RN, BS, MS
Barbara Wax, RN, AD
Gail Deterling, RN
Marilyn O'Connell, RN, BSN
Chris Lyons, RN
Nora Koller, RN, BSN
Leslie Wood, RN
Dorothy Spinney, RN
Nancy Berube, RN
Mary Burke, RN
Melissa Flon, RN, BS
Colleen Souza, RN
Claire Leonard, RN
Patricia Pingree, RN, MSN
Terry DeMille, RN
Kay O'Meara, RN, BSN
Pat Poworoznek, RN, BSN
Patricia Phillips, RN
Carolyn Lundeen, RN, BA
Ann Marie Donovan, RN, BSN
Janet Haught, RN, BS
Sheila Connolly, RN
Ellen McTiernan, RN, BSN
Kathy Andolina, RN, BSN
Emily Dunn, RN, MPH
Virginia Nickolls, RN
Sharon Rothwell, RN, BSN
Lynn Huehnergard, RN
Susan Keeler, RN
Michelle Metivier, RN, BSN
Carolyn Henry, RN, BS
Sally Guy, RN, BA, BSN
Sally Talty, RN, BSN
Virginia Minihan, RN, BS
Melanie Neville, RN, AD
Cynthia Ruiz, RN, BSN
Georgette Hurrell, RN, BSN
Debbie Gagliardi, RN
Mara Ruments Wermuth, RN, BS, MSN
Paula Dugdale, RN, BSN
Mary Rose Condon, RN, BSN
Mary Kate Rondeaux, RN, BSN
Bonnie Edmonds, RN